Indulge Your Way to Healthy

A 13-Week Guide to
Rewiring Your Brain
and Creating Sustainable
Lifestyle Habits

Donna M. Morin

*Kelly –
Thank you for being
such a light in
my life.
xo Donna*

Indulge Your Way to Healthy:
A 13-Week Guide to Rewiring Your Brain
and Creating Sustainable Lifestyle Habits

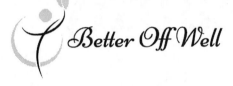

Better Off Well

Published by Better Off Well Publications.
www.betteroffwell.com

Designed by Andrea Reider
Andrea Reider Design
andreareider.com

Illustrations by Daryl Enos

Cover Photography by Jennifer Gresham
http://www.blinkbyjen.com/

ISBN-10: 0-692-85798-2

ISBN-13: 978-0-692-85798-4

Editor's Note: This book contains the thoughts and opinions of the author and is in no way intended to be a replacement for appropriate medical advice. Consult a physician for medical symptoms that may require diagnosis and treatment.

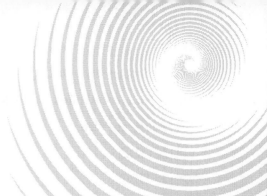

Contents

Part I

Part II

Part III

For P-Dad and Marny,
who helped to birth this project.

Acknowledgments

I TOOK THE longest to write this part because I am certain to forget someone. For this reason, I want to start by thanking all of my friends and family. Know that each of you has touched my life in some way and therefore changed it. Thank you for trying out recipes when I ask you to; it helps me so much.

Thank you to Julie Garland, Sara D'Allesandro, and Rose Sawyer for reading through my completed manuscript and making me feel like I had really produced something good. Even before that, I have Karyn Bilezerian and Tracy Dorcil to thank for reading first chapters, then encouraging me to keep going. It feels good to be supported.

Jennifer Gresham has fine photography skills, and knows how to make this camera-shy gal feel more comfortable in front of a camera. Daryl Enos, I LOVE your illustrations and I feel very lucky to be a recipient of your talent.

More than that, I thank you for being the inspiration that reminds me it's never too late to go after your dreams.

Kristi Marsh, your veteran advice is priceless to me, and our time together with the Savvy Women's Alliance has taught me so much. Thank you for your kind words and support.

For the members of the Magic Storymakers who taught me how to bring words to life and most of all, how to persist even when you don't feel like it...thank you.

Andrea Reider, thank you for sticking with me through edit after edit after edit, and responding to my emails within minutes. That meant a lot to this first-time author.

Julie Kinney, thank you for offering your beautiful book store as the place to launch this book. I couldn't think of a better place for that to happen.

So grateful for my readers at Better Off Well, who let me know that what I post is important to them and who consistently share their own tips. You may not realize how much you inspire and motivate me every day.

Many thanks to my clients, present and past, who have taught me that real, authentic health is about so much more than food and exercise.

For my son, Max. Thank you for being patient when your mother had to work and for always being willing to try my newest recipes. Even the disasters.

Frank Smith, you are the rock to my roll and I need that in my life. Our Friday night routine is grounding. Thank you.

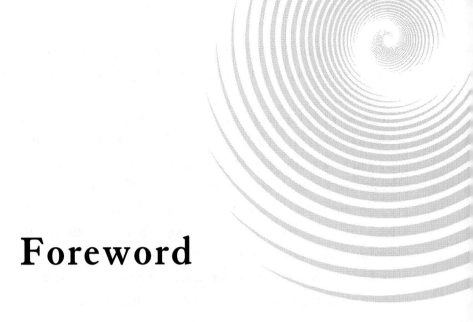

Foreword

THE WORLD is shifting. Can you sense it? Just by opening this book, you too are preparing for change.

At the beginning of my journey, I focused on my home and my one-acre in order to make tackling this world of eco-health more manageable for me. It took time to adjust to changes but I soon felt good about my changes. I was empowered by switching out products and enchanted by the foods my family started to eat.

Once I had grown comfortable within my own one-acre, I branched out and encouraged change among friends who were curious. Instead of feeling powerless, I found my voice, and began educating at women's conferences and encouraging our government to support legislation - with the end goal to protect our inalienable right to health.

Initially, I set out solo on a journey intent on building a new lifestyle, but actually ended up building an army. What started as a team of women supporting and following my heart, led to the founding of the Savvy Women's Alliance; a non-profit whose mission is to provide all women a safe place to listen, learn, and share about topics related to eco-health. Some women are at the beginning of their journey, looking to change out one product at a time, and others are ready to change the world. Savvy provides the forum for us to step out of our comfort zones and encourages other women, showing it doesn't have to be difficult. It doesn't have to be expensive. And you are never isolated.

So where are you on the journey? And why are you here? The road we start walking often leads us down many beautiful and unplanned paths. Often we think we are doing it for ourselves. Because we *should*. We are *supposed* to. But the sweetest truth is this: when we gravitate toward healthier living, we are inadvertently doing it—as Donna states so beautifully: *"To save the world, really."*

The pages ahead will inspire and encourage you. Donna's voice is clear, gentle...peaceful. It's a beautiful collection of storytelling and smoothies, honesty and health. You may dog-ear pages in order to return to tantalizing recipes, but don't be fooled—the heart of this book is a sharing of love.

A love for life. A love for health. For each other and our world.

Enjoy the journey,

Kristi Marsh
Author of *Little Changes*
Founder of Savvy Women's Alliance

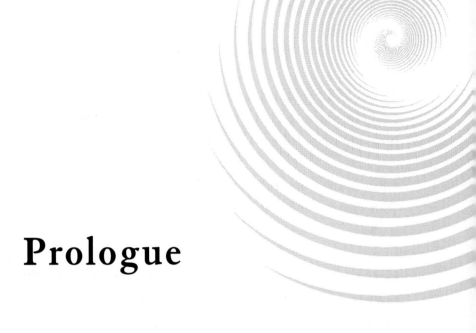

Prologue

Tell me, what is it you plan to do with your one precious life?
— MARY OLIVER, *The Summer Day*

COLUMNIST Katharine Whitehorn once wrote about extreme altruists, "You can recognize the people who live for others by the haunted look on the face of the others."

I only heard the quote this morning for the first time and yet I realized immediately this is why you are only reading this book now. You see, when I began writing this book six years ago, I was writing it for you. I began this book as a way to help you.

To save the world, really.

So I froze a few pages in.

The book-in-progress sat inside my laptop for years, never really in progress, though I would admit to writing a book now and then, fully aware of the lie that was.

I had heaped upon myself the burden of responsibility for your change, and rather than bear such a heavy load, I put it away.

Only through the inspiration of such authors as Elizabeth Gilbert and Steven Pressfield was I able to pull this work out again and dust it off. I realized the true purpose of this book would be in the art of writing for myself. Therapy for me. If you get something out of reading this book, I am grateful, but the only way I can finish is to recognize that the work is merely a selfish need for expression, and that this is okay.

It's not perfect, or award-winning. It's conceptual and quirky, but it's all mine and it represents my journey, the steps I've taken so far to get me to where I am today.

Once I was able to let go of this idea that my objective was to change your life, I was free to succeed or fail. That might be the best kind of freedom there is.

And so it is with you, Dear Reader. You are free, every day and every minute, to succeed or fail. Both will happen in your lifetime; both have already happened. But you have no one to answer to except yourself. Not your mother, or children, or spouse, or journal, or bathroom scale. It's you that you live with for every moment so any change you make from here on out should be just for you.

Do it so you get the most out of this one precious life.

Do it for you.

A Little History

I just. couldn't. breathe.

My body was tight. Adrenaline coursed through my veins. I wanted to inhale. Deeply. Badly. So badly. But couldn't.

It was 35 years ago, yet I still recall that day at Karen's house like it happened last week.

"Just calm down and breathe," Karen's mother said.

She was trying to help. I sat at her oak kitchen table, slumped over, shoulders tight, grasping for every breath. My friend next to me staring wide-eyed, quiet.

It was an asthma attack, and I'd done something nobody prone to severe asthma is ever supposed to do. I allowed the liquid in my portable inhaler to run dry. That sweet nectar that relaxes swollen muscles around inflamed airways was gone. Yet between each shallow breath I jammed the white, plastic tube into my mouth and squeezed anyway, hoping at least for fumes.

What I didn't realize then, thank goodness, is that I could have died that day. Every year, according to the Asthma and Allergy Foundation, more than 62,000 people are admitted with asthma attacks. Every day, 9 people die.

After what seemed like infinity, my father arrived with a new inhaler. I tearfully shoved it back into my mouth. Within seconds, I was breathing again.

Exhaustion, a few days of chest and abdominal pain, and irreversible lung scarring were the only consequences for my 14-year old body. Could have been worse.

This was often my life growing up. Diagnosed with 43 allergies at age 8, there was always something to trigger my asthma. Or maybe it would be the swollen eyes and congestion that would keep me indoors in spring and fall. Forget visiting friends with cats. Even being near people who had animals was a challenge because of hairs and dander that lingered on clothing.

At 22, I was admitted to the hospital for pneumonia. Too stubborn to see a doctor, I was hauled off by my parents who'd had enough of my incessant coughing and gagging that persisted for over a week. The nurses were excited to have me on their geriatric floor; I guess pneumonia was more typical for that age group than my own. The doctor later told my parents that a couple more days could have meant death for me; my lungs were so clogged with phlegm.

Like a cat with nine lives, I seemed to defy death once again at 30, when I was diagnosed with cervical cancer. Caught early enough, it only required two surgeries and a good chunk of my cervix to remove.

All was good after that until the day I sneezed in my class-room—and threw out my back. I was 33, and spent the rest of that day teaching hunched over. After months of pain, two MRI's, and a visit to a back doctor and physical ther-apist, I begged for a prescription that might help me walk upright again. I took the giant orange pills (now banned because of risks for heart abnormalities) faithfully, and life was bearable.

Until the times it wasn't. On one particular three-hour trip to New Jersey, we stopped for lunch. I sat too long. Barely able to get myself out of the car, I waddled to the restroom. Most poignant in that moment was the older woman with the long silver hair in the flowered print top and the mauve bag clutched to her body, who cruised right on past me.

For me, this was reality. Life. And I was cranky as hell.

I never questioned what I might be doing to cause any of it. I didn't know I *could* cause any of it. Or perhaps more importantly, I didn't realize I might be able to prevent all this.

Don't eat too many sweets so you don't get cavities.

Avoid too many calories so you don't put on weight.

Stay out of the sun to avoid skin cancer.

Don't smoke cigarettes or use recreational drugs because they can destroy your life.

Common advice I heard since I was old enough to hear. Outside of that, what could I do? Allergies and asthma were random, bad-genes kind of luck, and back pain happens to everyone when you get older. Cervical cancer? Well, meet the wrong guy in college and you get what you deserve.

That was the extent of my health knowledge. This was my pattern of thinking.

I had no power. Powerless.

Or so I thought.

Life-Changers

PART I

Something happened in 2004 that changed my life. Saved my life.

My son was born.

Having a baby is a profound experience. Having a baby come into your life through adoption is a whole different kind of profound. I felt almost unworthy of this gift and perhaps even guilty to accept.

I saw my son on the day he was born.

Swaddled in a thin white hospital blanket with blue and pink trim, his dark eyes looked straight into mine with something that looked a lot like confidence. It was as if he were saying, on that very first day, *So you are the one I am here for.*

His father and I left the hospital a few days later with a borrowed car seat holding a baby. As we moved through the automatic doors, I looked back over my shoulder, expecting somebody to stop us. We were taking a baby. *Do you people realize we are walking out of here with a baby?* But no one stopped us. A few lessons in diaper changes and swaddling and apparently we were good to go.

But we were not. Good to go, that is. We were clueless. Frightened. My years of babysitting did nothing to prepare me for the task of motherhood.

As I looked down on that sleeping peanut during the first of many sleepless nights, I knew I owed the woman who gifted me this boy my solemn commitment. In that silent moment, I pledged to do everything within my being to transform this tiny bundle of vulnerability into a healthy, responsible man.

But there was a problem to overcome first.

Growing up with a mom who didn't allow me near a stove, I knew convenience best. That conveniently led to an extra 25 pounds around my hips once I hit my 30's.

At the time, I ate vegetarian, but I was really a box-etarian. Much of what I ate was ripped open, tossed into the microwave, and ready in minutes. I owned only a few cookbooks, including, *Microwave Meals in Minutes*. A can opener was really the only cooking tool I owned.

That began to change after my son was born. It was then I started to read books that taught me how important food was for the proper development of a body.

Huh.

I read that plants—vegetables, fruits, nuts, seeds, beans—had micronutrients that were found, through scientific studies, to work magic in various complex functions that are performed every single day. These functions help our bodies to thrive and keep us from getting sick or becoming diseased.

Huh.

I started to turn over boxes and read ingredients. A coupon clipper whose only criteria for food was a cheap sale price and what tasted good, I never read labels before. I trusted the front of the package. If it said "vegetarian", it must be good for me. If there was a picture of fruit on the front, bonus! If the chocolate pop-tarts were advertised to have fiber, it was a miracle health food.

I didn't realize how many of my favorite foods were full of sodium, chemicals, and other processed ingredients. Then I would nuke the hell out of my nutrient-deficient food, making it even more nutrient-deficient. Which meant when all was cooked and done, I was eating tasty… crap.

Only now do I realize that was why most of the time I felt like crap. Granted, at that time I was existing in new-mom sleep deprivation fog, but the back pain, lethargy, asthma attacks, and frequent colds were not helped by my diet.

How could I have known that? I knew vegetables were "good for you" but what did that mean? The tomatoes in the sauce on my enchiladas counted, right? The vegetables they put into my veggie burgers? Food was something I ate because it tasted good and I was hungry, though the latter reason wasn't always necessary. I never considered food as fuel, never mind a kind of medicine.

While my son toddled around the train table at the bookstore, I pored through cookbooks. I wanted to make real meals for him, but would need help. Sure I could follow recipes with pasta and Velveeta and soy sausages, but now I wanted to know how to chop vegetables and what to do with them. I discovered brown rice, avocado, and sweet potatoes. Then there was asparagus, artichokes, and beets. Eventually there were collard greens, kale, and Swiss chard.

When my son entered preschool, I hit the gym three mornings a week. That was a whole new kind of motivation for me. My new food habits gave me energy and my new gym habits trimmed a few of the pounds I had tucked away. What's more, I began to enjoy cooking. It felt like art. Granted, I was copying someone else's work, but a finished, prepared meal was something to be proud of. And I was. After all, I'd never done it before.

Then another man entered my life and changed it.

Life Changers

PART II

Just as my son joined my life through adoption, so too did I join my family through adoption. I met my birth mom while in college and it seemed apparent right away that my personality was gene-driven. Where my adoptive family was generally quiet, stoic, and reserved, I was often annoyingly talkative, emotional, and opinionated. I loved to laugh and tell bad jokes.

Sally's smile was one of the first things I noticed. It was big, and her eyes lit up whenever she talked. Our first conversation together could have been far more awkward but Sally made me feel comfortable. Her laugh was like a musical hug.

Over the next few years, I asked a lot about my birth father. Sally realized this missing piece was a void I needed to fill, so she reached out to a friend who knew a friend who knew my biological brother. The son of the father we had in common.

The second time I met Paul, we were sitting in the backyard of our father's home in upstate New York. I put my son down to crawl on the plush, green carpet of a lawn, and my brother said to me, "I wouldn't do that; our father uses chemicals on his lawn."

Now keep in mind this was still the early stages of my lifestyle changes. At this point, I was discovering the benefits of eating real vegetables and playing at the gym. I still assumed everything sold on store shelves was perfectly safe and that there was no way it would be there if it were not. Somebody was watching out for us.

So when my brother spoke those words of caution, I gave him a giant mental eye roll, hauled my son back onto my lap, and thought, *Great, my brother is a wacko.*

Over time, I would get to know my brother better. I would learn that he liked to write, as I did. He would introduce me to Johnny Cash and composting. He would call me just to ask how I was doing, which was not something my childhood family usually did. He was sentimental, too. Score one for genes again.

Paul would also be the one to introduce me to this idea that not everything sold on store shelves was necessarily safe. Turns out, this wacko was the publisher of a successful magazine, host of a cable program about gardening and landscaping, a consultant for organic lawn care practices, and a well-sought after speaker, activist and writer driven by his own personal health story with lawn chemicals.

Since we've met, he's gone on to publish two books, an award-winning documentary, and is currently Chief Sustainability Officer of a huge project in Maryland, turning over 200 acres of lawn into a symbol of organic sustainability.

Wacko.

Life-Changers

PART III

I would be remiss if I didn't make mention of the book that started the ball rolling for me. Since then, there have been many others and I will provide you with a listing on page 45 of this book.

It was during one of my bookstore treks that I picked up a type of book I never had before. In the pages of *The Green Smoothies Diet*, Robyn Openshaw taught me about the power of the plant. About compounds inside of plants that served important functions in the body. Through her story, I learned food can heal. Thus began my smoothie-making venture, and starting my days with the kind of leafy greens that never before entered by vocabulary, much less my body.

My blender at the time was a beat-up Cuisinart, and calling it a blender is probably being generous. But there I was, churning up fruits and greens, carrots and avocados.

My first smoothies were chewy, but I drank them anyway. Robyn was that convincing.

It would be a year later, as I sat at my computer freelancing an article, that I would have an epiphany. I had not used my asthma inhaler in over a year, nor taken back medication. Over the coming years, I would also realize how little my allergies bothered me and how little I sniffled through cold season.

Mind-blowing.

My new lifestyle choices began with a desire to lose a few more pounds, prevent future illness, and to be a healthy role model for my son.

Nobody had ever told me that asthma could be reversible, or improved, or prevented. Nobody ever told me that my allergies didn't have to be as bad as they were. There was never mention of diet when I went to the doctor crying with back pain.

That is the reason for this book.

I want YOU to know what I did not. I want you to understand that you have more power than you may believe.

You can heal your body. You can feel good.

The extent of healing will be different for each one of you. It may depend on factors like how committed you are, your age, and your personal health struggle. But I am confident you have the power to make improvements, no matter what.

You. Have. Power.

Here is what else you need to know.

You can't teach anyone what they don't want to know. That's a big one to remember. If you are reading this book because you want to make changes in your own life or in the lives of your young children, then I am really excited for you and I hope that much of this book resonates with you as others have for me.

But if you're looking to change a partner, a friend, or someone in your family, stop and take a deep breath. It's not that you can't influence positive change. You can! But the best way we influence change is by modeling it. As Mahatma Ghandi said, "Be the change you wish to see in the world." Each of us is on her own path and as difficult as it may be to watch ones we love travel their own, we can only support when it's asked for and continue working toward our own most authentic self.

Perhaps the most important lesson I've learned that I want to impart to you is that living a full and healthy life has to do with more than food. You can eat broccoli all day, or take supplements, or try every cleanse you read about, but if a relationship is failing, you hate your job, or you feel a void that can't seem to be filled, then none of that will make much of a difference. At least not for long.

That is why this guide was created. Food is important and the way we feed our bodies will impact the energy needed to make lifestyle changes in the first place, but it's the emotional, mindful, and spiritual changes you make that will determine how sustainable your new habits are.

What's Happened To Our Food?

Let's start with the most obvious. Whether we realize or not, we have an intimate relationship with food. We reintroduce it to our bodies multiple times every day. It's important, then, that we understand how it's changed.

I see what is happening to some very beautiful people today. Men and women who work long, hurried and stressful days, only to come home to meals that deplete their bodies of the very nutrition they need to keep their energy levels up. Mothers who would do anything for their children, but make almost no time to do anything for themselves, which includes eating food that would help them to feel great. Children who are often sick with sneezes and sniffles, or worse, because their eating habits do not provide their growing bodies with the nutrients they need to ward off illness and the fiber they need to ensure a healthy gut.

Like me for most of my life, I don't think everyone understands what they are up against in our culture today. Industry has turned food into a technological frontier. What began as part of the feminist movement and a celebration of freedom from the constraints of domestic life has turned into an experiment and we are the lab rats. One popular food flavoring company describes itself as a "leading supplier of customized, technology-driven food and beverage solutions…"

I don't know about you, but the idea of my food being driven by technology feels wrong. Call me old-fashioned, but I want to eat the kind of plants that start from a seed, that grow with sunlight and rain, and that are harvested by another human who went home and made dinner with the same food.

I know this might be unrealistic, given our world population these days and the need for methods that don't always require soil since we are destroying more topsoil every year, but there are changes to our food system that I can't get behind.

Genetic modifications, chemical flavoring, colors, preservatives, pesticides, added fats, salt, and sugar have changed our food so that it is far from the food our human bodies evolved to eat and is often simply edible, not really supplying our bodies with the tools they need to thrive, never mind to just function properly.

The corn in a frozen corn dog, for example, did not start as a seed that was a descendent of an earlier generation of corn, as was typical in farming practices not so long ago. It was likely purchased in bulk from a bio-engineered supply of corn seed, meaning that the seed itself was injected with an insecticide meant to kill insect predators. The seed is also a "terminator", making it impossible to be used by future generations, forcing the farmer to purchase new seeds each year and making the concept of "heirloom" vegetables ever more rare.

Food scientists work in labs creating just the right balance of chemical flavors, salt, fat, and sugar that will entice the hell out of your taste buds and dopamine receptors in the brain to keep you coming back for more of their product.

The individual slices of cheese "product" in the plastic wraps that still look like plastic after they come out of the plastic? They are less than half actual cheese and more milk by-products, additives, preservatives, and food colors. Hence, the name "cheese product" on the package.

Food has become an exact science, meant to manipulate our senses, taste buds and pleasure hormones, while growing the bottom line of billion dollar food companies, and we are at its mercy as long as we continue to remain stressed, over-scheduled, and uninformed.

There are ways to change all that. We don't have to partici-pate as lab rats; we can reduce the stress in our lives; we can become informed, and we can live happier lives as a result. I have my degree in education, certifications as health coach and in stress reduction, and I write. I am not a doctor and I do not pretend to play one on TV. I do, however, have years of research and anecdotal evidence. I know what has worked for my clients and what hasn't. Most importantly, I know what has worked to help me reclaim my own health.

We are always on a journey. This one precious life is ours to live, which means growing and learning all the time. One step in front of the other keeps us moving forward. With this book, I hope you will see how much fun it can be to move toward a healthier lifestyle, one indulgent step at a time.

What's Different About This Book

I wanted to write this book because I think most people see positive lifestyle changes as challenging, dull, and even unattainable. Changes can definitely be that way if we dive in head first, become obsessed with scale numbers, and expect to see immediate improvement. The changes I made have been gradual, over the course of a decade, and even longer than that if you include my stride into vegetarianism.

I am big on baby steps. Just like a toddler has to first cruise the furniture and then high-toe her way to the next safety net, so too, do we have to start where we are and move as far as we are comfortable if we want our changes to become habits and part of a new lifestyle.

The first step has to be with your mindset. This is NOT a diet. Diets don't work. Not long-term anyway.

Diets require sacrifice, counting calories, and a never-ending internal battle of the wills. The word *diet*, as we have come to know it, represents something opposite of what you will learn in this book. Diet is one four-letter word I never want you to say again. Do not drop the D-bomb anymore. Unless, of course, you are referring to your diet as the foods you eat.

What makes this book different from other self-help diet books is not only that it's not a diet book, but that it's a book that focuses largely on changing you from the inside out. If you practice each of the steps in here, you will begin to notice a shift in how you feel about yourself. I think that's where most diet plans fail. Too much emphasis is placed on changing you from the outside in, or there is no focus on the "in" at all.

Instead of thinking a healthy lifestyle has to be difficult, picture yourself baby stepping your way into it. Every time you do something for yourself, it's an indulgence. It's a way to pamper your body so your body will pamper you back. Indulge yourself each week by learning something new and applying it to your life. Don't follow the steps in this book consecutively if that doesn't work for you, but do choose at least one new step every week so you keep moving. Think of this as homework for your New Life course and treat it seriously.

You can do this. You picked up this book for a reason, so I know you're ready to start. Each of us is in a different place in our life's journey, and no matter where you are, it's okay. I was a mess for most of my life; I just didn't know it. Whether you are stuck in your own mess, or are already well on your way to creating a better you, let this book be your guide to getting you and keeping you on the path you were meant to be on.

The Indulgence Plan

Okay, so here we begin what I call the Indulgence Plan.

Why Indulgence?

Because an important first step in any lifestyle change is mindset.

If you think of these changes as a new and different adventure, as something you GET to do for your body, you will be far more likely to stick with them.

There are never sacrifices when it comes to our health; only investments.

Honestly, indulging is what these steps are going to do for your body, for you. If you follow the plan, you will be indulging yourself—body, mind, and spirit—in a way that you may never have before. You deserve that, don't you?

It's time to get the most out of this one precious life.

Ready to get started?

Say yes.

WEEK ONE

Indulgence #1: Change your bulbs!

What??? The first tip in a book about creating a healthier me is to change my freakin' light bulbs? I think that's what you're thinking, but hear me out. I'm not talking about replacing every bulb in your home. Just the ones in your bathroom, or wherever it is you get ready in the morning.

Find ones with a flattering glow that allow you to see your own special glow. Avoid fluorescent and compact fluorescent bulbs, as they are the least flattering. Look for LED bulbs that are listed as "warm glow" or "soft white". A "bright white" label can work, too, as that is most like sunlight. Avoiding the blues is key to avoiding morning prep blues. They tend to highlight any perceived imperfections.

Of course, the ultimate goal of this book is to have you feeling great about yourself so that you love the image in the mirror, in any light, but we're human. We have a tendency toward self-criticism. Right now your Inner Troll might be controlling more of your thoughts than you prefer. So let's start with flattering light, shall we?

The bulbs I used to have picked up every line and microscopic pimple on my face. You know that microscopic pimples become large and ugly pimples if you dig and pick. And digging and picking makes you late. Which then stresses you out.

It's a terrible way to start the day.

Use light that flatters. You will leave the house on time and feeling better about yourself.

Have you met people who feel good about themselves? Who present with true, authentic confidence? They are a pleasure to be around, and no matter what they look like, they are beautiful people.

Indulgence #2: Read a label.

The method I once used to buy food was

A. What was on sale?

B. Did I like the taste?

That's it! I never questioned the safety of my food. How could it be sold to me if it wasn't safe?

Today I know differently. Corporate interests play a HUGE role in our government and decisions are often made that protect those interests before they protect ours.

Now it's your turn if you're trusting in the same way I did. Read a label on a food product in your home. I don't mean the nutrition label where you probably check the calories or fat content. Move your eyes further down and peruse the list of ingredients.

Are there more than five? Do you recognize them all? Throughout this book, you'll learn a little about some of the ingredients you might be finding on the side panel. For now, just notice. Read before you buy. Any surprises?

Indulgence #3: Drink a lemon.

Not a whole one. Start your mornings with a warm cup of water and squeeze of a slice of lemon. Warm lemon tea is like a hug. Honest.

Perhaps more importantly, a number of studies have found the flavonoids in lemon help to suppress oxidation (or "rusting") in our bodies, help to support weight-loss, and support our livers in the detoxification process. Your liver is the ultimate in multi-taskers, performing more than 500 functions, but it's most important job is that of detoxification, so any help we can give is important.

Most of my clients who start their days this way claim that doing so allows them to be more regular, and trust me, dropping a poop load in the aquatic bowl every morning is one way to help you feel lighter and super energized!

Be sure to brush your teeth after drinking (or eating) citrus as the acid can wear away the enamel on your teeth.

WEEK TWO

Indulgence #1: Avoid the left side of the bed.

Ever heard that expression about waking on the wrong side of the bed? That wrong side is the left side. If you believe in superstitions, anyway, which apparently the ancient Romans did. Thank goodness I am not an ancient Roman or I'd be screwed.

No matter what side of the bed you get out of in the morning, make sure it's with intention. If I wake and the first thing going through my mind is all I have to get done that day, I'm likely to feel tired and drag myself up and out. Or bury myself back under the covers. I will be more likely to focus on what doesn't go right that day.

On the other hand, if I open my eyes and tune in to the song of the birds, or the silence of dark winter, say "thank you" for being alive another day, or set an intention like "I have all that I need to be happy today", it makes a huge difference. Could be the 20 seconds that change your day.

So this week, pay attention to how you're waking and change it if you need to.

While we're on the subject of bedroom routines, I have to mention the importance of sleep.

Scientists have long been baffled about the purpose of sleep. Evolutionarily speaking, the need for hours of unconscious or sub-conscious presence doesn't make sense in light of potential danger lurking in the dark during our hunter-gatherer days.

But we do understand there are benefits. You don't have to be told how a full night of quality sleep makes you feel. More focus and productivity, healthier choices, and more energy often follow a good night of shut-eye. On the other hand, a lack of sleep affects hormone production, depleting energy stores and even messing with our satiety signals so we often eat more.

A fascinating animal study from the University of Rochester published in 2013 found that sleep may have even more importance. The cerebrospinal fluid in which a mouse brain floats during the day (as does a human brain) appears to be a cleanup system for the brain, much like the lymphatic system works in the rest of the body. While we sleep, this fluid flushes out toxins that may be linked to brain fog, memory lapse, mood swings, headaches, and seizures. More studies are needed to see if a lack of quality sleep could also be linked to Alzheimer's or other neurological disorders, because a brain that doesn't have time to flush out toxins will instead accumulate them, potentially leading to disease.

Do you feel refreshed when you wake in the morning? If the answer is yes, and you don't have a hard time falling or staying asleep, that is fabulous. Count your lucky sheep.

If, on the other hand, you're having a hard time getting to sleep or falling asleep, try this:

Make sure you have a soothing bedtime routine. Try a few minutes of deep breaths, meditation, or gentle stretching before you get into comfortable pajamas and complete your routine. A contemplative kind of book—not a thriller or cliff hanger—or a wellness magazine is often a good choice for bedtime reading.

Keep technology out of the bedroom. Try to place your phone away from your bed, your alarm clock turned away from you, and the TV out of the room.

Run a diffuser with sleep-inducing lavender essential oil (or whichever you prefer) while prepping for bedtime. I have one that turns off on its own so I fall asleep to the soothing scent and the gentle trickle of water.

Avoid eating a couple hours before bedtime, or at least high-fat foods that require extra work from your body. When your sleeping body does not need to focus energy on movement or digestion, it can apply that energy instead toward maintenance and healing.

Avoid caffeine after 3 pm. It can take up to 7 hours before the full effects of caffeine wear off.

Check with your doctor or do your own research to see if any of your medications could be responsible.

Indulgence #2: Learn something new.

Richard Branson, founder and CEO of the Virgin Group, says he sees life like the university education he never received. Every day presents an opportunity to learn something new. It can be as grand as signing up for guitar or language lessons, or as simple as memorizing a new word and using it throughout the day.

Tittle.

There's one for you. It's what you call the dot on a lowercase "i" or "j". Try using that one in a sentence today.

Connections between our brain cells, called synapses, are eliminated if we don't use them and sets us up for early dementia. The brain has about 10 million cells, and each is important for controlling bodily functions. Keep it strong by taking a new route to work, buttoning your shirt with a different hand, memorizing a poem or a favorite quote, learning a new dance, or having a Bananagrams throwdown with the family tonight.

Decide today what you'd like to know more about and find a way to make that happen.

Indulgence #3: Plank

You've probably seen it already. The plank is one of the simplest moves you can incorporate into your day anytime and almost anywhere. The move isn't easy, and that's what makes it so special, because this one move engages so many of your muscles, including core muscle groups, which are responsible for maintaining good posture and a strong back.

If you don't have a lot of time for muscle toning activity right now, then a few minutes of planking will begin to get your body into a good place.

Imagine your body is a wood plank, and your plank is somewhat parallel to the floor. You will look as if you are on the upside of a pushup, but no pushing up is required. Simply hold in pushup position for as long as you can. Be sure your body is straight, with your butt tucked in so it's not up in the air.

Make it a little more challenging by resting on your forearms and again, holding a straight plank position.

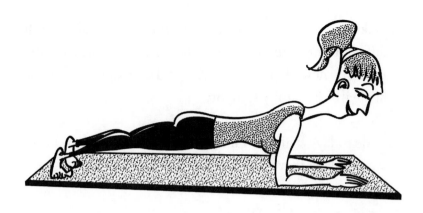

Perform the plank every day, twice a day, and watch how it begins to tone your body and make you stronger. Chart your progress. Dr. Oz says you're a rock star if you can hold a plank for a minute, but don't get down on yourself if ten seconds is the most you can do for now. It takes time to build muscle groups that haven't been used in a while.

I like to move into a downward dog position when my body has gone into high vibration mode and I need a rest. Then I go back to planking one more time. The plank has become a regular part of my morning gym routine.

WEEK THREE

Indulgence #1: Pottie All the Time!

Indulge *me* for just a moment, because we health coaches love to talk us some poo. Uncomfortable a topic as it may be for some, it's important.

One of my first clients years ago was a beautiful mom of five little ones. In our first conversation she told me she wasn't hitting the porcelain throne every day. Why?

Because she didn't have time.

Yep. This beautiful, selfless soul wasn't even taking the few minutes for herself to perform that all-important daily function. But I am sure she's not alone. I bet there are more of you out there doing—or not doing—the same thing.

I used to think I was a rock star on those days I didn't have to go. How convenient that was. But listen up. Poop happens. It has to. Every day. Once is good; twice is better. Third time—as plant-friendly author and actress Alicia Silverstone would say—is bonus.

Poop is made up of fiber, dead bacteria, live bacteria, dead cells, excess protein, toxins, and mucus from the lining of our intestines. Blech, I know. Most of it is stuff our body no longer needs and if it sits too long in our colon, the toxins can be re-absorbed and that can set us up for some major health problems.

So you truly must release the poop portal every day. Indulge yourself.

I kid you not; there's a poop chart, called the Bristol Stool Scale, developed at the University of Bristol in the U.K. and it was designed to classify human feces into seven categories. The seven types of stool are:

1. Separate hard lumps, like nuts (hard to pass)

2. Sausage-shaped but lumpy

3. Like a sausage but with cracks on the surface

4. Like a sausage or snake, smooth and soft

5. Soft blobs with clear-cut edges

6. Fluffy pieces with ragged edges, a mushy stool

7. Watery, no solid pieces. Entirely Liquid

You want to order up a #3 or a #4 when you hit the john. #1 and #2 mean you need some plunging, a.k.a. more fiber and water. If you've got time to read the paper while you sit on the throne, something is wrong. Go ahead and read the paper, but save it for the couch. Poop time should be short and sweet.

On the other hand, feces shouldn't be splashing out like water from a faucet. #6 and #7 are signs you may have an infection or other illness, which can be serious if it continues. More than half of our body weight is made up of water, and all cellular functions require water, so losing a whole lot of it into the toilet requires immediate attention.

Abnormal poo is a sign that something is not right within, so if you're not hitting the throne every day or you're hitting it every hour, be sure your fiber and water intake is at optimal levels and have a doctor check your gut flora. A probiotic, elimination diet, or other medical intervention may be in order to help restore balance.

Indulgence #2: Take a hike!

For real. "Forest bathing", or as the Japanese call it, *shinrin-yoku*, has been shown to increase our cancer-fighting white blood cells if we do it consistently. Studies have found that hiking is associated with lower risk of colon and breast cancer, and it may positively defer other types of cancer as well.

People who hike regularly are less affected by stress, have a healthy cardio-vascular system, better muscle tone, lower cholesterol and triglycerides, lower weight, better sleep, and decreased chance of depression.

So find your closest patch of trees and start moving among them. Bonus points if you stop to hug one.

Indulgence #3: Affirm Yourself

How many times in the last few hours have you reminded yourself of how beautiful you are? In the last week? Month?

If the answer is close to never, get out a piece of paper. Write, in large bold letters…

I AM BEAUTIFUL

Post it by your mirror so you see it every day. Dr. Christiane Northrup suggests that you talk to yourself like you would your best friend. "Hey, you look great today! Love that out-fit. Is that a new scarf?"

If right now your Inner Trolls are telling you not to do this because you are not beautiful, then make the sign even bigger.

Your Inner Trolls are those negative voices that creep into your head when you're not paying attention. They are the Dark Force. They represent the Resistance that you feel anytime you try to do something to make yourself a better person. They will tell you to sleep in when you want to get up early to hit the gym. They urge you to have the second piece of cake when you were satisfied with one. The trolls will do everything to convince you that you are not good enough as you are.

You do not have to let the Trolls win, but recognize them, identify them, and understand that they creep back in every day, so affirm yourself often.

Your desire for a healthier you has to start from a place of self-compassion.

Seems crazy, but this concept might be the most difficult for many of us. It was hard for me for many years. It's been difficult for many of the women I've worked with.

If you have a hard time affirming that you are a beautiful person, or with finding beautiful qualities about yourself, dig in. Ask yourself why. What kind of messages have you received in your life that makes this part so difficult? The answers may take a while to come but they are important to ponder.

Love yourself just as you are right now. Cellulite, zits, unwanted hair and all. Until you start to do this, you will always find flaws with yourself, no matter how much weight you lose or toned your body is. Taryn Brumfitt, director of the film, *Embrace*, was blown away when she overheard the women in her body building group, with their thin, muscular frames, still finding fault with their own bodies. It led to the creation of her documentary that spans the world in search of positive body messages for women and Taryn does a fabulous job showing us why these messages are so important. I highly recommend if you need a little body love inspiration.

None of us is perfect, but it is within those imperfections that authentic lies. The Japanese have a concept of *wabi-sabi*, which nurtures all that is authentic and real and imperfect. It values age and wear and the quirks that make objects unique. We need to apply *wabi-sabi* to our own selves and value those characteristics that make each of us unique.

Why be upset with laugh lines when they mean you have spent a lifetime laughing? Why be afraid to express your interests when those very interests make you interesting? Why care about cellulite on your legs if you are fortunate to have legs that can take you wherever you want to go?

WEEK FOUR

Indulgence #1: Build Your Tribe

If you've been following this plan week to week, we're nearly a month in on this journey. This next Indulgence is truly critical so I ask that you take it extra seriously.

The times my clients have experienced the most lasting success have been those where they have built a tribe of support around them. You can't go this alone. You are amazing and you can do amazing things but there are going to be times you will forget why you're making the choices you are. You will find yourself steeped in emotions or surrounded by others who are not in the same place as you. And no matter what, unless you live in a yurt on a mountaintop, you are living in a culture of fast and processed, material and self-interest. A support system will make all the difference.

If you already have a friend or two interested in making this journey with you, you're off to a great start. Don't be afraid to ask. Somebody else might be looking for a wellness buddy, too. Family members who are supportive will make your steps easier to follow. Not everyone is lucky enough to have this kind of support, but do not despair. There are lots of ways to build your tribe, and they work just as well.

Hire a personal trainer or health coach and meet on a regular basis.

Find a wellness group through Meetup.com.

Join a yoga class and enlist the help of your yoga teacher to keep you on track.

Like to hike? Check out www.outdoors.org or www.hiking andbackpacking.com.

If mountain biking is your thing, check out www.single tracks.com.

Purchase a subscription to a magazine so you receive regular reminders and tips and the feeling that you are not alone in your journey. Check out experiencelife.com, www.vegetariantimes.com, www.motherearthnews.com, or motherearthliving.com. I recommend avoiding magazines that focus solely on the physique. Living a healthy lifestyle cares less about external beauty and more about energy, vitality, self-growth and self-awareness. And when you have those things, you've got external beauty.

If social media is part of your day, find pages through Facebook, Twitter, and Pinterest that offer recipes, tips, and inspiration.

Start a book club using a book that focuses on wellness. Open it to the public and hold your meetings at the local library. Consider these books...

Big Magic, by Elizabeth Gilbert

Crazy, Sexy Diet, by Kris Carr

Clean, by Alejandro Junger

Eat Dirt, by Dr. Josh Axe

Living a Charmed Life, by Victoria Moran

Little Changes, by Kristi Marsh

Madly in Love with Me, by Christine Arylo

Positivity, by Barbara Frederickson, PhD

Revive, by Frank Lipman, MD

Radical Remission, by Kelly Turner, PhD

The Four Agreements, Don Miguel Ruiz

The Gifts of Imperfection, by Brene Brown

The Green Smoothies Diet, by Robyn Openshaw

The Life-Changing Magic of Tidying Up, by Marie Kondo

The Power of Now, by Eckhart Tolle

The War of Art, by Steven Pressfield

The Willpower Instinct, by Kelly McGonical, PhD

What are You Hungry For? by Deepak Chopra

When Food Is Love, by Geneen Roth

Wherever You Go, There You Are, by Jon Kabat-Zinn

Wild, by Cheryl Strayed

Indulgence #2: Laugh

This week I want you to laugh. Hard. Pretend to laugh if you have to. Studies have found children laugh way more than adults do. Not that we needed a study to tell us that. When was the last time you had a good belly bust? A time that your cheeks cramped from giggling? Remember how great you felt after? Relaxed, rested, full of joy.

Dr. Madan Kataria was so impressed with the health benefits of laughter—lowered blood pressure, improved immunity, decreased stress—that he created what is now sweeping the country as Laughter Yoga.

The concept is simple—laughter can be induced without the use of jokes or outside influence. This is at least one time where it's okay to fake it. Heck, it's encouraged that you fake it. I can laugh like I've just flown over the cuckoo's nest all by myself and my body will still receive all the benefits.

Of course, it's way more fun to fake laugh with a bunch of friends because it soon turns into real laughter. You probably don't want to try this while standing in line at Target lest people start running away, but hey, if they do, you won't have to wait in line anymore.

Healthy Snickers…

"If at first you don't succeed…then skydiving is definitely not for you." –Steven Wright

"Why do they call it rush hour when nothing moves?" – Robin Williams

"Some people create happiness wherever they go; others whenever they go." –Oscar Wilde

"First the doctor told me the good news: I was going to have a disease named after me." –Steve Martin

"I am constantly amazed by Tina Fey. And I am Tina Fey."
–Tina Fey

"Never, under any circumstances, take a sleeping pill and a laxative on the same night." –Dave Barry

"Make-up can only make you look pretty on the outside but it doesn't help if you're ugly on the inside. Unless you eat the make-up." –Audrey Hepburn

"My fake plants died because I did not pretend to water them." –Mitch Hedburg

"My grandmother started walking five miles a day when she was 60. She's 97 now and we don't know where the hell she is." –Ellen Degeneres

"I find television very educational. Every time somebody turns on the set, I go into the other room and read a book." –Groucho Marx

"Trying to be happy by accumulating possessions is like trying to satisfy hunger by taping sandwiches all over your body." –George Carlin

Indulgence #3: Grateful-ize Your Life

Google "The Power of Gratitude" and you'll come up with hundreds of different pieces.. When Oprah Radio aired, its host Richard Losier said that by becoming practitioners of gratitude, we attract positive, vibrational energy into our lives. Sounds new age-y and incense-burning, I know, but think of it this way: when we begin to focus on all those things going right in our lives, we focus less on what isn't. So we feel less like the world is beating up on us.

When we recognize all that is going right, we feel lighter... happier, content, at peace. When we feel at peace, we want to take care of ourselves and show concern for those around us. When we are happier, healthier, and concerned about others, we attract more people to us who bring their own brand of positivity. When there are more positive people in our lives, there are more opportunities for positive encounters and thus our opportunities for happiness are increased.

You don't have to write anything down, but many people find keeping a gratitude journal has made a big difference in their lives. Start this way: at the end of each day, write down three things you are grateful for. Try to vary what you write, and be specific. For example, instead of writing that you're grateful for your children, you might write how you loved that joke your daughter made up or the way your son looks when he sleeps.

There are days you will not be grateful for your children and instead you will be grateful for a particular room in your house where you can lock the door and breathe alone for a few minutes. Point is, when you hone in on details, you are likely to notice those details often. And little things make a big difference. Over time, you will not only practice gratitude, you will live gratitude.

END OF DAY GRATITUDE

Now I lay me down to sleep
The wonder of today I keep
Green blades of grass
A clear blue sky
Laughter in my son's brown eyes
A garden full
My belly, too
Berries red and berries blue
Friends checking in to say hello
Arms and legs that make me go
A brand new book
With crisp, clean pages
More words of wisdom from the sages
What I don't have matters not
Because what I have is quite a lot.

–Donna M. Morin

WEEK FIVE

Indulgence #1: Introduce Yourself to a Stranger

Say hello to a pomegranate. Or an artichoke. How about a plantain, endive or spaghetti squash? Ten years ago, I'd not had either of these. Would not have been able to identify either in a lineup. Now I find them in my meals often. On purpose!

What foods are you missing out on? You may think you don't like beans, but there are more than twenty different types of edible beans just in the U.S. and each has a different flavor and nutritional purpose.

It's time to be adventurous. If you can't be adventurous with your food, just think of where else in your life you may be holding yourself back!

Scour the produce aisle or farmer's market and commit to trying something you never have. Type the new and exciting item into the search bar at www.epicurean.com to find a way to prepare it. Stop missing out on the little pleasures of life.

Indulgence #2: S—t—r—e—t—c—h

As I wrote this stretch of the book, I lay on the floor of my new-to-me, tiny post-divorce apartment in one very eloooooongated stretch. It was necessary because I typed away on the floor, not having found a desk yet. If I didn't stretch, I'd have been ambling around with a walker by week's end.

I remember times I attempted to touch my toes and couldn't make it past my knees. There were days any attempt at bending was a painful proposition and simply out of the question. Today, I make sure to stretch often because it makes a difference in how I feel.

There are so many benefits to doing it.

Stretching...

- *lengthens muscles*

- *reduces muscle tension caused by stress*

- *enhances muscle coordination*

- *increases range of movement in joints*

- *improves blood circulation and energy levels*

- *provides pain relief*

- *improves posture*

- *offers a greater sense of well-being*

When you're stretching know that a little discomfort is fine; pain means stop.

Stretch both sides. A healthy lifestyle includes balance, and that applies to stretching as well.

A couple stretch tests you can try at home:

Lift one arm up and bend at the elbow, reaching down your back. Bend your opposite arm and place it behind your back. Try to touch the fingers on your other hand. Repeat but change arm positions. Can't touch? Then make arm and shoulder stretching a priority during your daily routine so you can inch your way closer.

Now stand tall and slowly bend at the waist, reaching for your toes with your hands. Note how far you can stretch. Now take a tennis or squash ball and, on a carpeted surface,

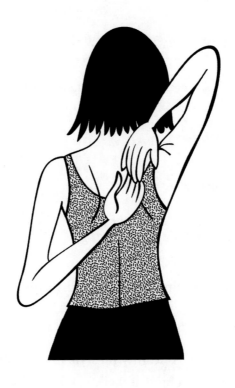

roll the ball under each foot for one minute, stretching your fascia tissue. Try the bend again. Notice any difference? If you are far from touching your toes, sign up for a beginner's yoga class, or find gentle stretches on-line that you can add to your daily routine. It's that important to a healthy, active, and pain-free future.

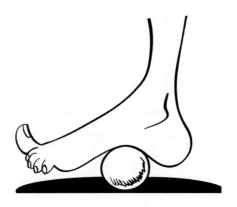

Indulgence #3: Beat Down Sugar Blues

When I was younger, I thought the reason to avoid sugar was to keep all your teeth. While that's likely still the case, I think most of us try to avoid sugar these days because we believe it will make us fat.

It can.

When our bodies take in too much sugar, whether in the form of too many calories or too many simple carbohydrates (think breads, pasta, pastries, and candy), the pancreas has to pump out more insulin so all that sugar can enter the cells through receptors and be used as energy. At some point in this mega insulin shoot-out, however, the pancreas goes on strike. From that point on, it either refuses to release more insulin, or the insulin it does release doesn't do its job. The sugar then stays in our blood, which sets us up for a slew of potential health troubles, including weight gain, diabetes, cancer, and Alzheimer's.

At that point, excess sugar may be stored as visceral fat, which is the kind of fat that takes up residence around important organs, keeping them from performing their jobs as efficiently as they might otherwise.

And there's still more that sugar can do. It can make us moody and blue, wrinkled and pimply, tired and lazy. Our skin is an organ, and so is the brain. Just like other organs in our bodies, they are affected by what we put into them.

But sugar can be highly addictive. It's been likened to crack cocaine in how it lights up the reward and pleasure areas of the brain for some people. Over time, the happy hormones associated with sugar consumption become depleted, so even more sugar is necessary to get the same effect, similar to a drug addiction.

So let's do this part in baby steps. The first step to beat those sugar blues is to become aware of just how much sugar you're taking in.

When you are checking those labels in your home or at the store, notice the sugar content. How many grams of sugar? Do you know how much a gram is? I didn't. In Catholic school, the nuns often warned that the U.S. would be switching to metrics any day so we'd better learn how to use metrics quickly.

Still waiting.

Until that happens, know that **4 g =1 tsp.**

3 tsp= 1 tbs.

That bowl of cereal with only 14 grams of sugar per ½ cup serving that you eat every morning? It has 3 ½ tsp of sugar per serving, which means you're probably starting your day with at least 7 tsp of sugar every day.

Say what?

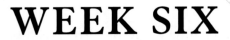

WEEK SIX

Indulgence #1: Schedule Time to Be SELF-ish

These days, you don't have to live in New York to be living on a New York minute. Most of us are consistently in a state of duress.

We drink coffee because we tossed and turned all night.

We text because we are too busy to talk.

We drive-thru because we have to get home, or to the ball field, the ice rink, another job.

We drink more coffee to get us through the end of the day.

We eat pizza or boxed food because we don't have time to deal with chopping.

We flop on the couch and stare at the TV because we're so exhausted from all that busy.

We watch something "mindless" and snack "mindlessly" because we're too tired to think.

We toss and turn at night because we overloaded on coffee.

Repeat. Repeat. Repeat.

We even wear this kind of schedule on our sleeves like a badge of honor. Clearly a fully scheduled life means we are doing important things, and so we feel important.

Why do we need so much mindless productivity to feel important?

I suspect at some level, we need it because this kind of busy feels like purpose. Were we to take time to examine our lives at a deeper level, we might actually feel the void that isn't being filled by all this rushing around. An over-scheduled life, in that case, leaves us feeling depleted instead of fulfilled so we turn to external sources, like caffeine, food, alcohol, sex, or retail therapy, to fill the void.

I'm going to bet that even our cave-dwelling ancestors knew when it was time to hang back and carve a stick or paint a buffalo on a cave wall. Yet very few of us today actually take time for ourselves. To meditate. To ask big questions. To express our creativity.

To just be.

Over time, this kind of consistent over-scheduling wreaks havoc. It's soul-crushing, really, but for now let's focus on what it does to our physiology.

Stress hormones interfere with many of our body's functions, including the production of hormones responsible for hunger regulation, digestion, and sleep. They deplete our immune system, and drain energy stores. A buildup of stress hormones like adrenaline and cortisol can cause brain fatigue and memory loss.

If we eat while stressed, our bodies convert more of the food we eat into fat.

I know what you might be thinking.

"Yes, this is my life, but I don't know how to do it differently. I need to earn money to pay for what we have and what we do. "

Or maybe you have many children with busy schedules, an infant, multiple jobs, an aging parent. Maybe this is just how life is right now.

I totally respect that. There is more here that needs to be addressed with other indulgences customized just for you, but let's start small.

If you need to be busy because life as it is for you now depends upon it, you need to take breaks. If you don't, you will not be productive for long. You will get sick, tired, and your creative process will be limited. Your mental capacity can only capacitate so much, so your mood will be changed. A depressed or irritable mood weakens relationships and that, in turn, creates isolation and potentially broken homes or failed relationships.

Time for yourself is clearly as important as the time you're punching on the clock, even a metaphorical one. Perhaps more so.

Because time to indulge yourself is so important, it must be scheduled. If you're the kind of person who's trained yourself to incorporate regular self-ish time, then pat yourself on the back and move on to the next indulgence.

For those who put off such time until tomorrow and tomorrow never seems to get here, then you have to treat it with the attention you would for any other health appointment. So go get your calendar right now....

...yes, now...

...I mean it...I'm waiting for you...

and now start jotting in your SELF-ish time.

A time indulgence doesn't have to be big. So let's start with a few small, easy-to-fit-in ideas.

Tea Time: when was the last time you sat for ten minutes with a cup of tea? I don't mean mindlessly sipping on tea while you update your way through Facebook or pay the bills. I mean really sitting, for ten minutes, warm cup in hand, tasting the tea, and having wistful thoughts. Don't you deserve ten minutes to yourself? And you get the benefits of tea. Green, white, and black teas are full of antioxidants and cancer-fighting compounds, but there are some delightful herbal blends that have body-balancing benefits as well.

Inhale on 3; Exhale on 6. You're breathing right now. You've been breathing since you started reading. And before that, too. More than likely, though, it was shallow breathing. And that's fine to keep us alive, but to get the true benefits of oxygen, we need to inhale and exhale with conviction. Like you mean it. Doing so clears our lungs of stale carbon dioxide to make room for that cell-replenishing oxygen. Try this everyday at least once, but especially if you're feeling stressed. Stop what you're doing, close your eyes, inhale deeply three times, as if you were filling up a bike tire. Count to 3 as you inhale and slowly release to a count of 6 as you exhale. Relax your shoulders while you're at it; they're likely attached to your ears.

Daydream. We've been told since we were kids that we shouldn't do this, but I say go ahead! Take a few minutes to stare out the window and imagine the possibilities. Where do you see yourself in a year? Five years? Where would you be right now if you could be anywhere you wanted? Who would be with you? Allowing ourselves to dream can be the catalyst to making those desires come true, so indulge.

Other SELF-ish Ideas:

- Hike in the woods with a friend or on your own

- Belly-dance or take a cooking class

- Book a massage

- Color

- Read poetry

- Write a poem

- Journal

- Sit in a book store café with a favorite book

- Watch an indie film

- Sit on a bench in the park and watch people

- Stare up at the night sky

Indulgence #2: Make Like Fred Astaire and Add A Little Ginger to Your Morning

Oh my, yes, that was corny. You may have figured out by now that I do, indeed, have a weird sense of humor. I've learned to be okay with it.

Growing up, I always loved old musicals. I never saw dancing and singing like that anywhere else. I still get lost in them today. Wouldn't this world be a much happier place if at any time during the day, people broke out in song and dance?

I picture myself gracefully lifted onto the checkout counter at Target by teen cashiers with hormonal acne while all other customers form a chorus of backup dancers and singers and big-band music blares from the speakers above, and I twirl and tap…

Oh, uh…ahem.

The ginger I'm referring to is the kind that looks a little like a brain cell. Grated fresh ginger makes a great addition to your morning tea, smoothies, juices, dips, and soups. Ginger has anti-inflammatory properties so it helps to douse the fire that exists within many of us.

When we are under constant stress and eating nutrient-deficient foods and lots of animal products, our bodies become acidic and inflamed, which creates a ripe environment for disease. Ginger's anti-inflammatory compounds, called gingerols, have the potential to reduce arthritic pain, ease post-workout aches, help with nausea, combat cancer growth, and keep colds and flu at bay.

So this week, pick up ginger and start twirling... I mean grating. Start grating.

Indulgence #3: Clean off your desk.

The eastern philosophy of Feng Shui views clutter as blockage of energy, or *qi* (chee). Ever noticed a difference in how you feel after you've carted those boxes of extra stuff off? You look into your closets and everything has a hanger. There is space in between each piece. The toys in your children's rooms found homes (and the idea that they will be returned to those homes after play time). Ahhh...you breathe. Your shoulders don't feel so heavy. Your energy is no longer blocked.

If eastern philosophy isn't your thing, think of it this way. When a home is cluttered, there is more energy expended. You need to find room for it, keep it clean and dust-free, and iron it before wearing because it was wrinkled from being crammed into the closet. Clutter = stress and that = a way to escape from the stress which often = food.

But here's the thing. For most of us, the idea of de-cluttering our homes is overwhelming. It's a task that will take days to complete, and then more days to haul off the stuff or send it away to good homes.

So don't do that. Vow this week to simply clean off your desk. Clean out a closet. Or the toy box. Maybe one book shelf. Most important, keep the areas of your home that you spend the most time in as clutter-free as possible.

Turn on your favorite tunes, make a cup of tea, and focus only on the project at hand. If you get into the flow and end up tackling the bedroom, too, then great. But the goal is only one part of the house. Keeping the task manageable will make it easier—and kind of fun—to get done!

Note: when you get to read Marie Kondo's Life-Changing Magic of Tidying Up, she will offer you a whole different approach. I loved it and—a year later—I'm still working on applying it.

WEEK SEVEN

Indulgence #1: Play detective!

You are smart. You know what foods are "good" for you and which are "bad".

It's intuitive.

You probably don't fall for the "real fruit" claims on the front of the toaster pastries—though I was a believer in denial for many years. What you might not know is that some of the foods you think are good for your body have hidden ingredients. When we consume foods like that, we sabotage our health and we don't even know it.

One example is the processed iced tea mix that I used to drink by the gallons and that I find in many pantries. While neither brand is a great choice because it's all sugar and chemical flavors, at least one popular brand promotes itself as being healthy. When you read the label, you find ingredients like aspartame, genetically modified corn syrup, six artificial colors (to make brown iced tea, mind you), and chemical flavors.

One client found sugar and MSG in her store-brand sunflower seeds. What the...?!?

Homemade Iced Tea Mix

One way to eliminate sugar from your life is by using better alternatives. Honey is still sugar, but local honey has added nutrients and natural antibiotic effects. Make your own iced tea so you avoid added chemicals, colors, and bleached cane sugar.

3-4 tea bags black tea

8 c filtered water

¾ c local honey

¼ tsp stevia

juice of a lemon

Steep tea bags in boiled water for 8-12 minutes. Add honey and stevia. Allow to cool, then add lemon juice and refrigerate. Serve over ice and with a sprig of peppermint, if preferred.

This week, clean out one shelf in your cupboards. Have your kids help you. Give them magnifying glasses and a highlighter. Look for ingredients from the list in the Appendix at the end of the book. See if you find any surprises. One of the most important steps in any journey toward a healthier lifestyle is simply becoming aware of what we're putting into our bodies.

Indulge in your future health by eliminating 5 food products from your home that contain artificial ingredients that do not serve your body.

Indulgence #2: Bust a Gut!

In week 4, I asked that you find a way to laugh, even if you had to force it. Even fake laughter provides benefits to our immune systems and helps to loosen tight muscles.

This week, I really want you to bust a gut. You know, that kind of laughter where you find it hard to breathe and your abs and cheeks actually hurt? I don't think we laugh like that enough, and I love that feeling after I do.

When did you last see a funny movie? I polled my readers and friends and came up with this list of suggestions for every kind of laughter preference.

Extra points if you watch with a friend who makes you laugh.

Funny Flick Picks:

Ace Ventura

Airplane

Bad Moms

Borat

Bridesmaids

Bridget Jones's Diary

Caddyshack

Date Night

Dumb and Dumber

Elf

Finding Dory

I Love You, Man

Love, Actually

Meet the Fockers

Monty Python and the Holy Grail

My Best Friend's Girl

My Cousin Vinny

Parental Guidance

National Lampoon's Christmas Vacation

Sausage Party

Super Troopers

The Secret Life of Pets

There's Something About Mary

Ted

The Blues Brothers

The Heat

The Other Woman

This is Spinal Tap

Trading Places

You Don't Mess With Zohan

Young Frankenstein

Indulgence #3: Walk the distance.

We've made it all the way to week 7 without me even mentioning moving your body. Not that it means this isn't important, and I really hope you're already doing that, but I know cram-packed schedules make hitting the gym difficult. And sometimes we find no pleasure in an oversized room lit by fluorescent lights and full of sweaty bodies standing in front of mirrors or pounding away on moving platforms.

If that's you, then forget about setting up a workout schedule for now. Let's just get moving. Our hunter-gatherer ancestors were always on the move, so they didn't need to hit the gym. You don't either, if you work activity into your daily life. Every fall I rake leaves, while leaf blowers buzz all around me. These days, it seems so archaic and absurd to be raking leaves, almost as absurd as it is to let machines do all our work for us and then pay for a membership to go exercise on machines when we could have gotten just as many benefits by not using machines to do all our work for us.

When I work in the yard, my heart beats faster and I swear I can feel my muscles grow a little. The next day, I feel genuinely worked out over my whole body.

That's really the secret to staying fit, trim, and energized. We simply need to work activity into our usual habits as often as possible. If you are running an errand in your car, this week park as far away as you can. Bonus points for walking to your destination, if that's an option. Move light furniture around your home. Scrub floors. Use the bathroom on another floor. If it's the stairs or elevator, start climbing. Two at a time even better. Exception made if you are headed to any floor in double digits or are hauling a grand piano.

Note: I believe the point of an escalator is to get you to where you need to go faster, not to give you a free ride. Climb the stairs on escalators, too!

Getting our blood pumping this way helps to strengthen our heart muscle, builds bone density, boosts our immune system, burns calories, and releases feel-good hormones that make us want to keep doing more feel-good things for our bodies.

Exercise isn't just for the gym.

WEEK EIGHT

Indulgence #1: Make Like
Sherlock Holmes

Ellen Degeneres once said, *Sometimes you can't see yourself clearly until you see yourself through the eyes of others.*

I believe striving to be the most authentic we can be is the key to inner contentment, difficult as that can be sometimes because our thoughts and actions are often molded by cultural norms.

To begin this quest for your authentic, make like a journalist this week and interview three of your friends about the latest hot topic: YOU. Find three good friends who are typically supportive of you and have been positive influences in your life. Ask them the following questions...

1. What are my best qualities?

2. How am I a good friend?

3. In what ways could I better nurture the person I am?

This activity will do two things. First, it's nice to be reminded of all that is good within us. Too often we allow ourselves to focus on mistakes and imperfections. Blame that on the Trolls again. Why wait till our bodies leave this Planetary Fish Bowl to hear all the nice things people think about us? (And I do believe we hear them.)

Now use these answers for a little introspection. What are your strongest qualities and which ones might you want to make stronger? How can you use these qualities to create the lifestyle you desire? If you're told you're funny, maybe you consider a blog or (eek!) performing stand-up so you can get even more people to laugh because lord knows, the world can use that. If you are tenacious and stick to your guns, then setting goals and making a plan to achieve them should work for you. Being trustworthy and authentic could make you a great candidate for coaching or counseling.

I think question #2 might be the most important because the answers are some of the most important pieces to the puzzle that forms the whole you. Some of the answers to this question may overlap with those in the first question, and that's okay. Preferred, actually. The qualities that make you a good friend will be the ones you'll want to put the most energy into cultivating.

Finally, take note of the tips your friends offer for self-nurturing. Treasure those nuggets. A little outside observation might be just the kick in the behind we can all use to start taking better care of ourselves.

Indulgence #2: D-U-M-P the H-F-C-S

HFCS—High fructose corn syrup: an un-natural sweetener derived from genetically-modified corn starch and found in many processed foods—cereals, cookies, snack bars, juices and soda—though food manufacturers are beginning to dump the stuff and you should, too.

How is taking something away indulging me? Great question. The answer is that by removing this one ingredient from your home, your body will be another step closer to living its fullest potential. That is an indulgence worth indulging in.

In week 5, I told you about sugar and how much of it we consume these days, on average. This week, let's talk syrup. Not the syrups like maple and molasses, or even honey. While those are sugars, and should be treated as such, each has its own nutritional benefit. High fructose corn syrup, on the other hand, has none.

According to some functional medicine experts like Drs. Mark Hyman and Josh Axe, high-fructose corn syrup has been found to not only be biochemically different than that of standard sugar cane, but also a potential factor in leaky gut.

Say what?

That's right. It's not only our bladders that can leak. The more accepted medical term is "increased intestinal permeability" but fewer medical experts are dickering over the term as it becomes more obvious that leaky gut is potentially linked to a number of today's chronic illnesses.

The lining of our intestinal tract is meant to be good and tight, so that no intestinal bacteria, toxins, or undigested food leaks through. While research in this area is still new, it's now believed that some medications, stress, particular chemical exposures, and processed food break down that lining.

In the case of high-fructose corn syrup, the unbound fructose molecules require more of our bodies' adenosine triptosphate (ATP) energy, the very energy used to keep our intestinal pipes from leaking. When our pipes start to leak, the body reacts and the resulting inflammatory response can exhibit in many ways, through gastro-intestinal trouble, headaches, lethargy, chronic pain, sinus infections, autoimmune disease, and more.

While it won't be easy to eliminate HFCS completely from your diet, making sure it's not in your own kitchen cabinets is a great first step to take.

Indulgence # 3: Tinker with the Thinker

Yesterday's Self-Talk: Why are these things happening TO me?

Today's Self-Talk: Why are these things happening FOR me?

When we view life's events as opportunities for growth—even the crappy muck stuff and especially the truly painful parts—then we keep moving forward. Playing a victim role gets us stuck, and stuck is not a good place to be.

This does not mean we need to "get over it" when something truly bad or tragic happens in our lives. It means we are gentle with ourselves, grieve at our own pace, but recognize that somewhere in this mess of a disaster is an opportunity to grow, to make our own lives better and maybe to enrich the lives of others in the process. This kind of thinking helps us to move through grief with power.

WEEK NINE

Indulgence #1: Post a Quote

I love to read inspirational quotes. They might be ones I stuck to my fridge or above my writing desk. Wisdom helps me grow and keeps me inspired to do what I am and living the most authentic life I can.

Find inspiration daily. It's necessary.

We don't stop laughing when we grow old; we grow old when we stop laughing. – Lao Tzu

People will forget what you said, people will forget what you did, but people will never forget how you made them feel. – Maya Angelou

Find out who you are and be that person. That's what your soul was put on this Earth to be. Find that truth, live that truth and everything else will come. – Ellen Degeneres

Be the change you wish to see in the world. – Matahma Ghandi

I'm thankful for failures. They teach lessons.
I'm thankful for challenges. They build character.
I'm thankful for what I don't have. It shows possibility.
I'm thankful for what I have. Too much would be a burden.
                                                    – Cliff Michaels

I think the purpose of a sunrise is to remind me how lucky I am to be alive another day. – me

Indulgence #2: Say Thank You

Saying thank you is probably one of the easiest ways to change a life. Yours.

All the bad news streamed daily through media can be soul-sucking. It has the power to leave us feeling powerless. Saying thank you to a special presence in your life is a way to take some of that power back.

Is there somebody you are grateful for? Maybe it's a friend who helped you out when you needed it, or a mentor, or a family member that you couldn't imagine life without. Hell, it could be your garbage collector, mail carrier, or librarian. I'm pretty grateful for all those people.

Once you've thought of the special someone you'd like to thank, find a notecard and start writing. It really needs to be written, old school, and sent via pony express. Doing it this way requires a little more effort and forethought, I know, but that's the point.

And trust me, once you've popped those kind words into the mailbox, you'll get this giggle of excitement in your body for the next couple days as you imagine the recipient when she opens your card.

Power restored.

Indulgence #3: Say Sayonara to Trans Fats

Just like removing high-fructose corn syrup is an indulgence for your health, so, too, is removing *partially hydrogenated oils*—or trans fats. They are typically found in fried foods, margarines, breads, cookies, pastries, buttered microwave popcorn, condiments, and even nuts and seeds. Packages that read "no trans fats" can still, by law, have trans fats in the products, so be sure to read those ingredient labels.

Artificial trans fats are created in an industrial process that adds hydrogen to vegetable oils to make them solid. They are inexpensive, provide texture and taste to processed foods, and allow for a longer shelf life. When first produced in the early 1900's, the harmful effects of these fats on our bodies were not known.

Trans fats not only increase our bad cholesterol (LDL), they lower our good cholesterol (HDL), which is like increasing the amount of garbage, while removing the garbage trucks. Extra fat (or lipids) circulating through our blood vessels can lead to more fat deposits and increase our risk for heart disease and some types of cancer.

The Federal Department of Agriculture finally removed it as an ingredient with "GRAS" status (generally recognized as safe) in 2015 and gave manufacturers three years to find safer alternatives. Until that time, it's up to us to be vigilant.

WEEK TEN

Indulgence #1: Balance a Book

Remember when you were younger and were told that the way to best posture was to walk with a book on top of your head? Go ahead and try it right now. It will be easier if you choose a hard-cover.

Note how you hold your body while you walk with the book balanced. Your back is a little straighter, your neck naturally elongates.

You walk taller. You feel lighter.

Why do this practice?

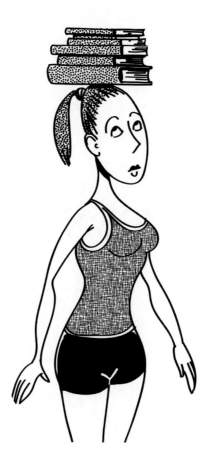

Because if you're like me and most other Americans who spend a chunk of their days staring at screens, it's likely your shoulders are hunched over and your abdomen muscles have taken a vacation.

Sitting for long periods of time every day is considered the new second hand smoking. When we sit for long periods of time, the dilation of our arteries shrinks, decreasing blood flow, including to our brains, which can explain why we feel so fatigued at the end of the day when all we've been doing is sitting.

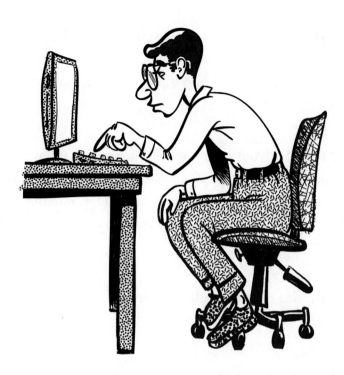

Sitting for long periods also impairs the body's ability to produce insulin. Since the job of insulin is to open the door to our cells so glucose can enter and be turned into energy, lowered insulin means that glucose stays moving through our arteries, increasing our chance for heart disease.

LDL—our "bad" cholesterol, is increased, and so are other fatty molecules. Additionally, enzymes responsible for breaking down fat decrease. Over years of sitting for long periods of time, bone mass decreases, especially in women.

Have I given you enough reasons to make sure you move through the day?

So starting now, wake up your ab muscles and let them know how much you missed them. Engage them to help hold your back in its natural spinal curve. Release your shoulders, keep your feet on the floor, and tilt your chin up a bit. Notice the subtle difference this makes in your energy.

Set a timer on your computer or phone so that you get up and move around every 40 minutes. Try chair yoga, stretch, walk while you're on the phone, encourage walking meetings, use the bathroom on another floor, take the stairs over the elevator.

In our office culture, sitting is often inevitable. The long-term negative effects don't have to be.

Indulgence #2: Look Sharp!

By now, I am hoping you've started chopping stuff up in your kitchen. If you haven't, here's where the fun starts. Time to purchase a new knife! Not something on sale that will turn your tomato to mush when you attempt your first slice, but a real, honest-to-goodness, Julia Childs would-be-proud kind of knife.

Honestly, I think one of the biggest impediments most people have to prepping real food is the inability to chop vegetables easily. I've worked in many kitchens where knives were too small, dull, old, and just didn't do the job. If chopping causes you to break a sweat you'll naturally avoid and turn to the pre-prepped processed stuff.

How do I find a good knife? I love using recommendations on Amazon, but here's what to look for when shopping for a good knife…

If you can, hold the knife. There should be a firm grip that feels comfortable.

The steel in the knife should travel all the way down the handle, unbroken.

Check the weight. I like mine to have some weight, without being heavy.

Be sure the handle is strong.

Quality knives use carbon steel blades because they sharpen well, but rust easily. High-carbon stainless steel is the next best option, and won't rust. If you're on a tight budget, a regular stainless steel blade is fine till you can invest more.

The cutting edge should run the full length of the blade, with no nicks.

Invest in a steel or sharpening stone to keep your knife working its best.

Indulgence #3: Breathe into the Chop

I'm going to stay on the topic of knives for a minute. Last week a friend told me he wanted to buy a vegetable chopper for me. This friend is all about efficiency, and he sees my daily veggie chopping routine as a waste of time. I disagree and explained this to him. For me, that time is all about slowing down.

While I chop, I might chat with my son about his day, listen to a podcast or soothing music, or simply relish in the quiet, feeling the smooth texture of a bell pepper in my hand and the way the knife slices clean through it.

So many of us today find meal prep to be simply a means to an end. The faster we get through it, the better. Often this kind of prep is symbolic of the way we live the rest of our days. Paying attention to the ordinary moments in the day adds a layer of richness we don't get otherwise. It's the kind of noticing that makes our lives more satisfying. When we don't get satisfaction from our lives, we often turn to food in an attempt to find it.

This week, prep for at least one meal by chopping something in silence or as close to that as you can. Use all your senses to be truly in the moment. Plan ahead for it so you can take your time, even if it's only one carrot. See if you notice a difference in how you feel once you've finished.

WEEK ELEVEN

Indulgence #1: Burn Fast!

Okay, you might again question my indulgence philosophy, but bear with me. Current exercise research has found that we can exercise for a mere 4½ minutes a day and still get the same benefits as a moderate hour-long workout.

That's right! 4½ minutes!

So what's the catch? Well, those minutes have to be pretty intense. You need to work your body up to a point where you can no longer speak. Think sprinting or riding really hard uphill on a bike.

This is often called HIIT, for high-intensity interval training and it's the philosophy behind 'functional fitness'. Scientists have found that our bodies work harder, burn more calories, and work more efficiently in improving our physical fitness when we work out this way instead of traditional, longer workouts that focus on one area of the body at a time.

Start with a couple minutes of warm-up, charge yourself HARD for 4½ minutes, then cool down for another couple minutes. Before you know it, you're adios-ing the other gym bugs who've barely begun to break a sweat.

Or maybe you're not at a gym, which is what's so cool about this workout. DO try this at home. The point is, our bodies were designed to move. We need to strengthen our heart muscle, keep our blood pumping so oxygen moves through the body and enters our cells, and improve bone density that tends to decrease as we age.

While you're at the gym, home, or on your lunch break this week, try the 4½ minute workout. If you've been putting off getting active because you don't have enough time, now you've got the perfect strategy for dealing with that.

If you don't like full-on hard core, can't-talk kind of exercise, don't stress. The benefits of a HIIT workout over traditional cardio are minimal, so if long-term, moderate exercise is more in your zone and you've got time for it, stick with that. The most important thing is to find activity that you enjoy, and keep changing it up so it fits your present lifestyle and so you don't get bored.

Indulgence #2: Ooh and Ah

This week, I want you to get really friendly with a piece of fruit.

Grab two plump strawberries, a couple orange slices, a sweet bell pepper, or your favorite kind of apple. Any fruit will work, really.

Begin eating the first piece of fruit. While you're eating, chat with a friend, yourself, check your email, or think of all those things you have to get done later.

Okay...finished?

How did that taste? Pretty good? Not sure?

Now take the second piece of fruit, or handful of berries, and pay close attention to the texture of the fruit. Notice the color. Feel it in your hands. Smell it.

Now take a bite.

Chew.

And chew.

And chew.

Chew more.

While you're chewing, close your eyes. Feel the texture of the fruit on your tongue. Feel where on your tongue you experience flavor.

What did you notice that time around?

It's amazing how much of a difference this makes. Studies have shown that mindful eating allows us to get more pleasure from our food, though we don't need a study to prove that. You just proved it yourself!

Mindful eating often results in consumption of fewer calories, less fat storage in our cells, better digestion, more nutrient absorption, and reduced chance for leaky gut. When we chew our food to a soggy pulp before swallowing, we increase the body's ability to absorb more of the nutrients in a plant's cellular walls. You get more bang for your berry, you might say.

Indulgence #3: Take Five.

Meditation is another piece of my self-improvement that has changed my life. While I've practiced off and on for a few years, it was a course in mindfulness-based stress reduction at UMass Medical that turned meditation into a habit for me. The MBSR Center in Shrewsbury, MA, was founded by Jon Kabat-Zin, author of the well-known *Wherever You Go, There You Are.*

Studies continue to prove the health benefits of meditation, including lowered blood pressure, fear, anxiety, and overall stress reduction. Meditation also grows the part of your brain responsible for focus, memory, learning, compassion and empathy. It helps us to be less reactive and more proactive.

Honestly, I believe if everyone in the world meditated, Earth would be an entirely different kind of planet.

Studies about meditation are still fairly new and scientists have not yet figured out the ideal amount of time need to get the most benefit. Anecdotal studies, however, have found that even ten minutes have made a difference.

I agree. There are days 10 minutes are all I can spare, yet even that helps. I still react less, and keep my cool more. I tend to misplace less, and ultimately get more done.

Honestly, if all you can make time for is to sit in your meditative position, then do that. Even just doing that shows a level of commitment to the practice and that totally counts.

The secret in retaining my practice has been to keep my practice scheduled at the same time every day. I meditate every morning for 15 minutes when I come back from the gym and most nights before I start my bedtime routine.

If all you can spare is 5 minutes this week, try it anyway. Just the practice of sitting still for a few minutes is benefit enough. As time allows and as you begin to grow and find a need for deeper meaning, you may make more time for meditation.

For now, just sit comfortably in a chair with your back upright a bit so your spine and hips are aligned.

Set a timer for 5 minutes.

Close your eyes.

Keep your feet grounded.

Focus on your breath.

Start by taking three deep Buddha belly breaths, expanding on the inhale and contracting on the exhale.

Breathe out all the excess air and imagine releasing all that isn't serving you.

All the worry. The self-defeating thoughts. Your to-do list.

Hold your body tall while you relax your feet, your legs, arms, shoulders, and jaw.

Return to your regular breathing.

As thoughts enter your mind, and they will, notice them. Try not to label your thoughts. Just notice.

Thoughts are like visitors; they come and go. You don't have to let them stay.

Imagine a broom gently sweeping the thought away, then gently return your focus to your breath.

Continue this process.

Take one final deep breath after the five minutes is up, and notice how different you feel.

Find time in your day when you can schedule in 5 to 20 minutes of meditation. The longer you stay and the more consistently you practice, the deeper you will be able to go and the more benefits you will receive.

Check my website (www.betteroffwell.com) for recorded meditations you may enjoy.

WEEK TWELVE

Indulgence #1: Say Thanks Before Chow.

It doesn't always happen. My son and I both have busy schedules. But as often as I can, I make it point to sit at the dinner table with my son and have some real chat time. As much chat as you can extract from a teen, anyway.

On these nights, we've started our meals by saying thanks for the food. Families have been saying grace for generations, but you don't have to be religious to make this happen in your home.

When we thank the farmer who grew the potatoes and the bell peppers, the migrant workers who harvested them, the trucker who carted the food across the country, and the worker at the food store who stocked the produce, we begin to understand just how connected we are to others on this Big Blue.

Indulgence # 2: Check your D

In the past decade, scientists have discovered just how important Vitamin D is to our bodies. Working with calcium and phosphorous to give us stronger bones and boost our immune system, D also plays a role in nearly every bodily function. Sun exposure causes our skin to produce Vitamin D, so a little exposure every day is key.

The Multiple Sclerosis International Federation released data in 2013, indicating a higher prevalence of MS in countries further from the equator. Vitamin D could also play an important role in the prevention of other diseases. In a study published by the National Institutes of Health in 2006, it was reported that Vitamin D supplementation may be a good way to help prevent breast, prostate, ovarian, and colon cancer.

The National Cancer Institute suggests a safe upper limit of 4,000 I.U.'s (international units) for adults and children over 8, though 1-2,000 may be all you need. If you've been feeling chronic fatigue, depression, anxiety, mood swings, or lack of focus, be sure you've had your Vitamin D levels tested as supplementation may be necessary.

Functional medical doctors like Christiane Northrup recommend 15-20 minutes of unprotected sun exposure every day during the summer, without skin burn, to help keep D levels at desired levels throughout the year.

It's a good idea to ask your doctor for an updated blood test and request that your vitamin and mineral levels be tested, in addition to the standard measurements. Because many people today lack diversity in their microbiome, it seems that essential strains responsible for the synthesizing and absorption of particular vitamins, like B12, may be missing and this will make a difference in your mood, energy levels, and your overall well-being.

Indulgence #3: Eat Bugs

Not the four-legged, winged creatures that you never want to find inside your shoes. I'm talking about bacteria bugs.

For most of our lives, we've been taught bacteria = germs = bad.

But picture this…your body is home for trillions—TRILLIONS—of bacteria. While it was once believed that our bacteria cells outnumbered human cells by about a 10:1 ratio, current science indicates the numbers are more even, and that a substantial trip to the Porcelain Throne could actually make us a bit more human for a while.

These bacteria are generally beneficial and play a role in multiple functions in the body, some of which we have yet to discover. They help us to digest our food, absorb nutrients, and produce hormones. Perhaps most importantly, they help to fortify our intestinal tract so that no undigested food particles or harmful bacteria slip through into our bloodstream.

While many of our bacterial critters could survive without us, we could not without them.

Unfortunately, scientists like Martin Blaser, author of *Missing Microbes*, have found the diversity of our bug village has decreased, and that appears to be linked to the rise in many chronic illnesses, particularly diseases traditionally characterized as auto-immune diseases like multiple sclerosis, Chron's disease, and Type 1 diabetes. Most recently, Parkinson's disease is among the latest to be tied to an imbalance in gut bacteria.

There is still much to learn about the ideal balance of strains, and it seems that our personal microbiomes could be as individual as fingerprints, perhaps making general recommendations more difficult. Early studies using both human and animal subjects, however, indicate that a high-fiber, plant-based diet could very well help to re-populate a healthy gut, as can avoiding high-sugar, processed foods.

Considering the correlation between the increase of fiber-deficient, nutrient-poor food in our typical western diet and the increase of chronic illness, asthma, hay fever, and food allergies, this makes a lot of sense.

In addition to high-fiber foods, it appears we get diversity benefits from a vaginal birth delivery, breastfeeding, having a dog companion, gardening, exercising, and living on a farm.

Eating fermented foods can also help to increase gut diversity as well. Quality, refrigerated pickles and sauerkraut, for example, encourage the growth of strains like *lactobacillus* and *bifidobacterium*, two common strains found in healthy people. Fermented foods are also a good source of vitamin K2, which is a form that appears to play an important role in heart health, brain function, strong bones, some cancer prevention, and bone strength.

As for taking probiotics, scientists seem divided. Some strongly recommend while others are more restrained, saying we still do not know enough about our bacterial ecosystem to determine which strains are ideal. Most seem to agree that to retain any benefit from probiotics, they must be taken consistently as the strains likely act more as traveling sales people than squatters taking up permanent residence.

I usually take a probiotic daily and many people I've worked with have noticed improvements when they have as well. A few have told me they notice how much better their medications work when they take probiotics. Not a surprise since scientists believe that our bacteria may be responsible for medication efficacy.

Another way to increase our diversity is to avoid doing things that lead to a decrease in our diversity. Overuse of hand sanitizers, over-the-counter and prescriptive medications, and antibiotics are high on that list. One day, antibiotics will be narrow spectrum and target only the problem pathogens rather than the broad spectrum antibiotics available today that kill off all bacteria, including our beneficial strains.

For now, use antibiotics only when necessary and with as much certainty as possible that a bacteria strain is being targeted, versus a virus, which will not be eliminated with antibiotics. Also, look for animal products that are antibiotic free as it is possible that even the miniscule amounts used in animal feed could be influencing our microbiome.

This week, take a step to ensure that your body is getting a daily dose of high-fiber foods including vegetables, beans, nuts, and seeds, as well as foods high in particular fibers our gut bacteria love, like Jerusalem artichokes, broccoli stalks, and green bananas.

WEEK THIRTEEN

Indulgence #1: Try a Cleanse

A cleanse can mean a lot of things, but I am keeping it simple here. If much of your diet at this point is clean—meaning that it's organic and homemade, using real, whole ingredients and lots of high-fiber produce, then already you are cleansing your body.

If eating this way seems out of the question at this time, then try it for a weekend. Plan ahead. Call it your "Cleanse Party" and ask friends to join in with you. Create a menu, rent inspiring documentaries, stay in your pj's or plan a hike in the woods. The point is…make it fun!

Another type of cleanse that works well for me a couple times a year is a sugar cleanse. I rarely eat anything made with processed white cane sugar these days, but I still indulge in dark chocolate, honey, maple syrup, and dried fruit. These are better forms of sugar, but still sugar and too much doesn't help a body.

Sugar, no matter what form, takes its toll on the body. Excess sugar produces inflammation, which breaks down collagen in the skin, making us look older. A study in 2015 also confirmed an earlier study from 1924 that found cancer cells do indeed consume higher amounts of sugar than other cells. When combined with body inflammation and exposure to carcinogens, excess sugar sets up our bodies as ripe real estate for cancerous tumors. When too much sugar circulates through the body, our bodies also store it as fat, often visceral fat, which is the kind that surrounds our hard-working internal organs, impeding their functions.

Do you feel sugar cravings often? Do you need a "little something sweet" after every meal? Are you turning to sweets every mid-afternoon to pick you up? Could you not even imagine making it through the day without sugar?

If you answered yes to any of these questions, a sugar cleanse will benefit you.

There isn't much to it. You don't have to make special meals or drink juices or give yourself enemas during this cleanse. You just have to abstain for 10 days to a month.

That may sound absurd and you may think you could never do it, which is why you need to do this. Your body will definitely throw a temper tantrum during this time. Some scientists even argue that certain bacterial strains in our bodies feed on sugar, and that sugar dependency multiplies these strains. They will not go down without a fight; they have changed your taste receptors and will send signals to your brain that could feel an awful lot like withdrawal.

Stick with it. Once you get over the temper tantrum hump, which is usually gone by the end of a week, you will find your cravings subside. Once that happens, and your body heals from the inflammation, you can reintroduce quality sugar on occasion.

When you're back to daily cravings, it's time for another cleanse.

Indulgence #2: Question Your Thoughts and Build Your Tribe

So many times we approach new health goals with an all-or-nothing approach. As soon as we start to slip on our commitment, we call it quits and label ourselves as failures.

Author James Joyce once said that mistakes are portals to discovery. Thomas Edison believed that failure was not actually failure, but the way you learn what not to do. JK Rowling, who was rejected often prior to Harry Potter success, said that failure in life is inevitable, unless you live life so cautiously that you might as well not lived at all.

To fail, therefore, is to live.

Failing does not make us failures, and that's where we get it wrong when we're trying to change habits. As soon as we miss a few days at the gym or gorge on Oreos at the family picnic, we internalize the mistakes as something having to do with who we are.

I can't do this.

I have no willpower.

This is too hard.

This is always too hard.

Sound familiar?

The good news is this: the kind of thought process you've been using to proclaim yourself a failure is simply another habit that you have the power to change.

The first step is to be aware of these thoughts. Listen to them as they move through your head. What are they telling you?

Next step is to question those thoughts. If you hear *I can't do this*, ask yourself what exactly it is you can't do. You can't stop eating chocolate when the 3pm craving hits? The more specific you can be, the easier it will be to address what exactly you are frustrated with.

Next, question if that thought is really true. Have the cravings always been so strong? Was there ever a time in your life where you didn't need chocolate at 3pm? You likely have lived through a time in your life where your habits were better, even if only a little. So that means you can do this; it's just that today you feel you can't.

Why not? What is happening today, or this week, that might be making the cravings particularly strong? Maybe the kids are beastly trolls this week, or you've had a lot on your plate with work or a sick family member. The weather may have been particularly gloomy or your best friend forgot your birthday.

Whatever the case, if you disown the fatalistic thought patterns and start questioning the specifics in any situation, you will start to see that you are truly not a failure, but human. That the issue is not permanent, but temporary and fluid.

Here's the other important piece, though. You have to keep coming back to the mat. It's a phrase I totally stole from yoga. In yoga, the literal meaning is to keep returning to your yoga practice so that you can retain all the benefits yoga provides. The bigger metaphor, however, is to consistently return to those elements of a healthy lifestyle that *keep you inspired.*

Going through a weight loss program and losing pounds is a fantastic accomplishment, but there will come a time when the weight loss will be difficult to maintain. We live in a culture that is fast and processed and unless we change our environment so that it includes daily support and reminders about why we are making the choices we are, it can be easy to fall back on old habits and thought patterns.

Remember to set your environment up so that it is supportive of your positive lifestyle habits. As I mentioned in Week 4, it's essential to build your healthy lifestyle tribe. For me, that means surrounding myself with people who live the kind of life I aspire to live. They could be friends, community leaders, yoga teachers, mentors through audio books, authors through print books, sages and their inspirational quotes to hang around my home, podcasts, classes, and retreats.

Form a book club and become a leader for positive change in your own community. It's a great way to meet people who aspire to live healthy lifestyles, too, and it provides a layer of accountability for you.

Set a long-term goal to accomplish something you've always wanted to try. It might be to hike a mountain, run a race, enter a triathlon, or bike a long distance. Working toward a goal like this, and eventually accomplishing the goal, is motivational and spurs you toward more similar successes

Failure may be inevitable, but if we learn from those times we failed, we have the power to create a support system in our lives that make the same failure less likely in the future.

Indulgence #3: Pretend You Died

I know. That sounded completely morbid in your head. It's funny how death is something we ALL have in common, yet it's the one topic most people avoid talking about.

Why is that?

I've started reading obituaries when I see them, even those of strangers. Why? I feel it's my small way of honoring the life of that person who passed on. Plus I like to read about people who made the most of their precious lives. We all touched lives, no matter if we think so or not, because we are all part of an interconnected web.

Through dying, people inspire me with their living.

For example, I loved reading about Shelly, who was always a helper and loved to laugh, or Burt, who was known for his silly gifts. There was Carol, who collected banjos, and Cicely, who knitted hats for most of her life and then donated them to shelters.

We don't have to do big things to influence this world in a big way, and I hope when I die that I am remembered for the way I lived.

That is the purpose of this indulgence.

Not to think about death, so much—though I think it's okay to think about death—but instead to think about how you want to live. What is it you want to do? Learn? See? Where do you want to travel? What do you want to accomplish? What, to you, is a life well-lived?

Pretend you're overseeing all that is going on once you've left your physical form on this planet. What is being said about you? Are you happy with that? If not, write out what you want to be said about you. Write your own obituary and plan your funeral. Try to take this indulgence lightly, but allow the end result to guide you in the decisions you make from here on out.

How will you get the most from this one precious life?

Indulge Recipes

The following are some of the recipes I've designed over the years. This coming from the gal who only knew boxed food and can openers for much of her life. The recipes are simple but very tasty. Please feel free to experiment with any dish and check out my cookbook suggestions below for more inspiration.

Make the kitchen your playground, your food lab, and have fun!

Favorite cookbooks:

Clean Eating Bowls, Kenzie Swanhart

Plenty, by Yotam Ottolenghi

The Complete Vegetarian Cookbook, by America's Test Kitchen

Thug Kitchen, by Thug Kitchen LLC

Veganomicon, Isa Chandra Moskowitz

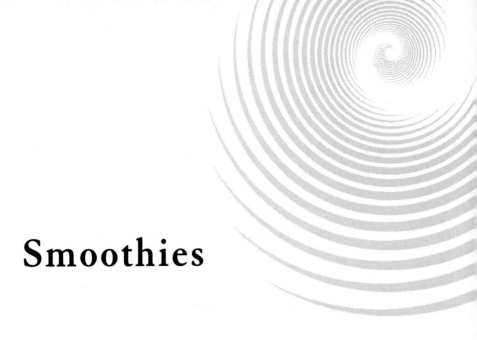

Smoothies

Power Orange Juice

1 banana, halved

2 Valencia oranges —juiced

1 tbs pumpkin seeds

1 tsp flax seeds

3 ice cubes

Blend until well mixed.

Pear Apple Passion

1 Bartlett pear, chopped

1 apple, chopped

2 c frozen greens

⅓ c plain yogurt

½ tbsp. flax seeds

1 c apple cider

3 ice cubes

Blend well until mixed. Add more water or cider, to get desired texture.

Wakeup Chocolate Smoothie

1 c frozen organic cherries

1½ c frozen organic strawberries

1 ripe banana

2 c swiss chard

1 handful frozen green beans (yes, really)

2 tbsp. cacao powder*

2 c coconut water

2 c filtered water

Blend until well mixed.

*Cacao powder is the raw, uncooked version of cocoa powder. Because it's not cooked, it has higher levels of minerals, like iron and magnesium, as well as antioxidants.

Breakfast

When I was growing up, breakfast cereal filled my morning bowl. Every morning. It got to a point I no longer had to think about it. Breakfast was as autonomous as breathing.

Inhale. Get out of bed. Exhale. Walk to kitchen. Inhale. Open cupboard door. Exhale. Pull out box....You get the point.

While I am not above indulging in a giant bowl of corn flakes now and then, that high-sugar processed stuff doesn't start my day any longer. If it did, I'd be needing another sugar fix mid-morning and a hot-fudge sundae for lunch. Back surgery for dinner.

So I've learned how to make yummy meals and snacks that keep me feeling great and fueled up. I am totally okay with snacking on plain old raw fruits and veggies, now too. My taste buds no longer throw temper tantrums when I do.

Berry Chia Pudding

Ingredients

1 bag organic frozen strawberries or 2 cups fresh

1 can coconut milk

½ cup almond milk

1 tsp vanilla extract

1 tbsp local honey (optional)

½ cup chia seeds

Directions

Chop strawberries so they are easier to blend. Pour milk into blender and add chopped strawberries. Blend well. Add vanilla and honey and blend again. Pour into glass Pyrex bowl or some type of storage container. Mix in chia seeds with a fork until all are blended. Cover and store in fridge. After 30 minutes, remove and stir again. Store overnight.

Note: you can eat this after an hour in the fridge, but the pudding will be thicker if you store overnight.

Overnight Breakfast Cereal

Ingredients

2 c oats

2 tbsp. chia seeds

3 tbsp. raisins

1 tsp. cinnamon

1½ c almond or coconut milk

Directions

In a pot with a cover, mix oats, chia seeds, raisins, and cinnamon. Cover with milk to about a half inch above the mix. Set in fridge overnight.

In the morning, you should have something that resembles hot oatmeal. If you want more liquid, go ahead and add more milk to your liking. Then add your favorite cut fruits, a sprinkle more cinnamon, nuts, and a drizzle of local honey or pure maple syrup.

PEANUT BUTTER BANANA OATMEAL

Serves 1

½ c steel-cut oats (highest in fiber of all oats)

1½ c water

1 tbsp raisins

1 heaping tbsp. peanut butter (with no added sweetener)

1 banana, chopped small

1 tsp cinnamon

Boil water and then add oats. Reduce heat to low for about 10 minutes. Sir in raisins and allow to simmer for 5 more minutes. The oats should have absorbed most of the water at this point, yet still have enough so oats are "creamy". Stir in peanut butter until mixed well. Remove from heat and add chopped banana and cinnamon.

Lunch and Dinner

BLACK BEAN BURGERS

Serves 3-4

1 can black beans (rinsed) or 1 1/2 cups cooked

½ c bread crumbs

¼ c flour

1 can tomato paste

1 tsp garlic powder

1 tsp onion powder

3 scallions, chopped fine

Smash beans with a masher in bowl, then add all other ingredients and mix. Don't be afraid to get your hands dirty and squish away. Form into patties of preferred size and cook in skillet till browned on both sides. Serve on greens or favorite whole wheat roll with greens, avocado, and tomato.

Hearty Chickpea Veggie Burgers

Serves 3-4

1 can chickpeas (garbanzo beans)

1½ c organic quick oats

1 lg. clove garlic

1 tbsp. chopped cilantro

½ tsp cumin powder

½ tsp sea salt

¼ tsp black pepper

2 eggs, beaten

Combine all ingredients in a mixing bowl until moistened. Form into burgers and place into heated, oiled skillet. Cook until browned on each side. Serve with crispy sweet potato fries and sautéed greens with garlic.

Chili with Basil and Kale

Serves 4

2 cans black beans

2 cans red kidney beans

2 cans garbanzo beans

½ jar seasoned tomato sauce (I like the 365 Whole Foods Italian Basil or Classic)

1 c vegetable broth (or add more tomato sauce)

1 chopped green bell pepper

1 chopped red bell pepper

1 small yellow onion, chopped

2 tbsp. fresh basil, chopped

3 leaves kale, de-stemmed and chopped

2 tsp chili powder

Add all ingredients to a large pot or crockpot. Simmer over medium heat for about 30 minutes. Enjoy with butternut squash quesadillas or chips and guacamole.

KALE & LENTIL BEAN PATTIES

Makes about 10 patties.

1½ c cooked green (brown) lentils

1½ c cooked (or 1 can) garbanzo beans

½ can (2 tbsp.) tomato paste

2 c kale, chopped small

½ tsp sea salt

½ tsp cumin

On a low-medium setting, pan-sauté the kale in a high-heat oil like grapeseed, organic canola, or high-heat coconut oil (note: extra virgin olive oil is not a high heat oil and should not be used for cooking). While the kale is cooking, mash the garbanzo beans with the lentils until almost all beans are smashed. Add the paste and seasonings and stir. When kale has cooked down, add to mixture and mix again.

Heat more oil (or vegetable broth if avoiding oil) in sauté pan. Form ¼ cup size handfuls of the mix into patties and gently drop into pan. Sauté each side until golden brown, flattening a bit as they cook. Serve over rice, quinoa, or with a salad.

Sweet Squish Burgers

Serves 4

1 sweet potato, cooked (about 1 1/2 cups)

1 c green lentils, cooked to slightly firm

1 happy chicken or flax egg**

2 tbsp. chopped red onion

1 tbsp. ketchup (no hfcs)

1/2 c crushed cornflakes (non-GMO)

2 tbsp. nutritional yeast

1 tsp. sea salt

1/2 tsp. ground black pepper

Oil for cooking.

**Egg only necessary if planning to serve as patties, as it provides some hold. If planning to use only as wrap filling, you can omit. Happy chickens means the eggs came from chickens that were truly free-range, preferably from a local farm, where chickens are allowed to scavenge and roam.

In large mixing bowl, use potato masher to squish sweet potato and lentils together till mostly mashed. In separate bowl, whisk egg (if using) and add to potato mixture. Add all other ingredients and mix well.

Heat oiled skillet on top of stove over medium heat. Squish mixture into patties about two inches in diameter OR saute mixture as is if planning to use solely as wrap filling (which I prefer). Serve on lettuce with chopped pickles, onion, tomato, and sesame seeds.

PINEAPPLE FRIED RICE

¼ cup raw cashews, chopped

1 cup frozen pineapple, chopped

1 red bell pepper, chopped

3 scallions, chopped

1 cup frozen peas

2 cups cooked brown rice

1 tbsp tamari (gluten-free soy sauce)

1 tbsp teriyaki sauce

extra virgin olive oil for cooking

Add chopped cashews to a large dry skillet on low heat and watch while you prep the other ingredients, stirring the nuts around until you start to see browning. Add a little olive oil to cover the bottom of the skillet and turn up the heat to medium-low.

Add pineapple and vegetables. Stir around for a few minutes until pineapples thaw and vegetables soften. Mix in rice and stir around for a couple more minutes. Add teriyaki and tamari, and turn off heat. Stir until well mixed. Taste. Add another tsp of tamari if you want a little more salty; teriyaki if you want a little more sweet.

VEGETABLE LASAGNA

Serves 4

2 boxes (gluten-free) lasagna noodles

1 20 oz. jar seasoned pasta sauce

3 c shredded carrots

5 c shredded spinach

2 c shredded arugula

2-3 c chopped tomatoes

"Cheese"

2 c whole blanched almonds (preferably soaked overnight)

½ c water

½ c lemon juice

¼ c extra virgin olive oil

2 tsp. thyme

2 tsp. rosemary

Blend all together in high speed blender until smooth and creamy.

Lasagna Directions

Boil noodles until al dente. Layer first set of noodles on bottom of 9 × 12 baking dish. Spread tomato sauce over noodles. Top sauce with a layer of almond cheese. (Tricky to spread. Not so pretty…but unless you've invited the queen to dinner, who cares?) Sprinkle carrots, tomatoes, spinach and arugula to cover. Layer again with noodles and repeat. Add final layers of noodles and top with remaining sauce.

Cook in oven at 420 degrees for about twenty minutes, until greens are wilted. Remove and serve.

Optional: top with dry-roasted pumpkin seeds for extra flavor and nutrition.

LENTIL JOES

1½ c coarsely chopped mushrooms

½ c chopped onion

½ c diced celery

1 garlic clove, minced

1 c cooked green lentils (till al dente, not mushy)

1 c chopped tomatoes

1 c tomato sauce with Italian seasonings*

2 tbsp. tamari (or gluten-free, non-gmo soy sauce)

2 tsp. teriyaki sauce

2 tsp. Dijon mustard

Sourdough bread or romaine lettuce for serving

In large skillet over medium heat, sauté mushrooms, onions, and celery for about 7 minutes. Add garlic and cook for 2 minutes longer. Fold in rest of the ingredients and reduce heat to medium-low. Cover and simmer for about 20 minutes. Serve ½ cup filling per bun or wrap.

*Can't find a sauce with Italian seasonings? Make your own with a tsp each of oregano, thyme, marjoram, rosemary, cumin, and sage, or whatever combination of those you have.

LENTIL SOUP

Serves 2-3

¾ c green lentils

1 1/2 c water

2 carrots, diced

1/4 c red onion

2-3 cloves garlic

2½ c vegetable broth

2 c chopped kale

2 tsp. GMO-free soy sauce

½ tsp. ground black pepper

1 tsp. curry

Pour water into a pot and add lentils. Bring to boil and then lower heat to simmer for about 15 minutes. Lentils should be al dente—somewhat firm to the touch. While lentils cook, saute carrots for a couple minutes, then add onions and garlic and saute for about 5 minutes more. Drain lentils when they are ready, and add carrot mixture.

Add chopped kale and vegetable broth. Mix should be covered by about an inch of broth, so use a little more broth if necessary. Bring back to a boil and then lower to simmer for about 10 minutes so kale can soften. Turn off heat, add seasonings, allow to marinate for five more minutes, and then serve. Season with sea salt to taste, if necessary.

Not-Tuna Salad

Serves 2

1½ c chickpeas (or 1 can, rinsed)

¼ c celery, finely chopped

¼ c red onion, finely chopped

1 tbsp. lemon juice

2 tbsp. mayonnaise

1 tbsp. dijon mustard

1 tbsp. parsley, chopped

1½ tsp. dried kelp powder

sea salt and pepper to taste

Use a masher to mash the chickpeas. Add celery and onions and mix. Add the rest of the ingredients and mix again. Easy!

Quinoa Burgers

Serves 3-4

2 c cooked quinoa

½ c gluten-free flour

2 happy chicken eggs, beaten

2 tbsp. Italian herb spaghetti sauce

⅓ c chopped onion

⅓ c grated, chopped carrot

2 heaping tbsp. chopped cilantro (or any other herb)

2 cloves garlic, minced

¼ tsp. ground pepper

1 tsp. turmeric or curry

½ tsp. sea salt

Whisk beaten eggs with gluten-free flour. Add cooked quinoa, sauce, onions, carrots, cilantro, and garlic. Mix together. Add remaining seasonings. Form into patties (will feel somewhat loose) and cook over medium heat, flipping after browned. Top with almond cheese, if desired, and serve with sautéed greens.

CAULIFLOWER COUSCOUS

1 head cauliflower

⅓ c raw cashews or almonds

1 heaping tbsp. nutritional yeast

1 tbsp. extra virgin olive oil

1 tbsp. local honey

Grind nuts in food processor till fine, and set aside in large mixing bowl. Chop cauliflower and pulse in processor till fine. Add to ground nuts, along with nutritional yeast, olive oil, and honey. Mix well. Add sea salt to taste.

At this point, couscous can be used in any way you might normally use this dish. Add whatever veggies you like.

Optional Vegetable Additions:

⅓ c corn

⅓ c edamame or lima beans

⅓ c chopped red bell pepper

⅓ c black beans

1-2 tbsp. chopped fresh basil

1 heaping tbsp. chopped red onion

1 tbsp. olive oil

1 tbsp. fresh lemon juice

Mix veggies with the olive oil and lemon juice and add to couscous. Serve right away or marinate in the fridge.

SUMMER SALAD

Ingredients for Salad

2 c frozen corn

1 c frozen peas

1 red bell pepper, chopped

2 tbsp. red onion, chopped fine

2 heaping tbsp. chopped basil

1 ripe but firm avocado, chopped

1½ c red cherry or grape tomatoes, chopped or halved

Pan sear corn and peas on low heat (no oil necessary), stirring occasionally. In large bowl, combine all other ingredients. Once peas and corn have thawed and there is a little brown on some of the mix, remove from heat and transfer to bowl also. Mix all together and top with a little sea salt or ground pepper, if desired.

INGREDIENTS FOR DRESSING

Juice from 1 lime

1 tsp local honey

Whisk together for about a minute till well mixed. Voila! Pour over salad and either eat or allow to marinate for an hour.

STUFFED SHELLS w/ QUINOA & CASHEW CHEESE

Serves 3-4

1 8 oz. box pasta shells*

2 c cooked quinoa

1 c prepared cashew cheese (not baked)*

2 c frozen peas

6 artichoke hearts, chopped

1 jar favorite Italian Herb spaghetti sauce (mine is 365 brand)**

Heat oven to 375 degrees. Cook pasta till just slightly al dente. (Be sure to test so they're not TOO al dente. They should not crunch.)

While pasta is cooking, mix quinoa with peas, chopped artichoke hearts, cashew cheese, and half the jar of sauce. When shells are done, rinse in cold water and place in prepared baking pan. Stuff spoonfuls of mixture into each shell. Pour remaining sauce over stuffed shells and place, uncovered, into oven for 12-15 minutes. (Gas stoves sometimes cook faster.)

Remove. Allow to cool for a few minutes, and serve. Garnish with parsley, if preferred.

*I use Tinkyada brown rice shells.

**See page 143

***If you don't have Italian Herb sauce, just add 1 tsp each of marjoram, oregano, parsley, and rosemary, and garlic powder.

Snacks or Appetizers

ALMOND CHEESE

1 c whole blanched almonds

¼ c water

¼ c lemon juice

3 tbsp. plus ¼ cup olive oil, divided

1 clove garlic, peeled

1¼ tsp. sea salt

1 tsp. thyme

1 tsp. rosemary, crushed

1. Puree almonds, lemon juice, 3 tbs olive oil, garlic, salt, and ½ cup cold water in food processor for a few minutes, until very smooth and creamy.

2. Use a spatula to slide mixture into small, shallow baking pan. (I used two small mini pie plates.)

3. Bake in oven at 225 degrees for about 25 minutes, or until "cheese" turns slightly brown on top. At this point you can choose to cool, then chill, or prepare seasoning to serve warm.

4. Seasoning: Combine remaining ¼ cup oil and seasonings and drizzle over cheese just before serving.

ARTICHOKE-SPINACH DIP

1 jar artichokes, 9-12 oz

2 c tightly packed spinach

1 tbsp. fresh lemon juice

1 tbsp. red onion, chopped fine

1 garlic clove, chopped fine

¾ c almond or cashew cheese

⅓ c nutritional yeast

¼ tsp. coarse sea salt

⅛ tsp. chili powder

freshly ground pepper, to taste

Drain artichokes and pulse in food processor till in small pieces. Steam spinach in a pan on top of stove for just a couple minutes, till slightly wilted but bright green. In a large bowl, mix lemon juice, onion, garlic, almond cheese, nutritional yeast, and seasonings. Add artichoke and spinach and mix again.

Bake in oven at 375 degrees for 15-20 minutes, until top is slightly golden brown.

Serve with baguette slices or gluten-free crackers.

Easy Power Truffles

¾-1 c raisins

¼ almonds, chopped

1 heaping tbsp. flax seed

1 tsp spirulina

1 heaping tbsp. cacao powder

Blend nuts and flax together for a bit until mostly ground. Add rest of the ingredients and blend until mixture starts to slow and clump. If too dry to squish mixture into balls, add another tbsp. of raisins and blend again.

Serve as is or roll in shredded coconut. Freeze for a few minutes, if desired.

Hot Chocolate Decadence

Serves 2-3

2¾ c So Delicious unsweetened coconut milk

3 heaping tbsp unsweetened cocoa powder

⅔ c pure maple syrup (Mrs. Buttersworth doesn't count)

1 tsp pure vanilla extract

pinch sea salt

⅛ tsp stevia (optional)

On low heat, add coconut milk to a saucepan. If cocoa powder is clumpy, sift into milk and whisk until mixed. Add maple syrup, vanilla, and sea salt. Taste. Not quite sweet enough? If that's the case, sprinkle the 1/8 tsp of stevia and continue to stir until simmering and ready to serve. Garnish with cinnamon or peppermint sticks.

Tomato Mango Salsa

3-4 c of fresh tomatoes, chopped

½ c fresh or frozen corn (drained)

¼ c red onion, chopped fine

½ c fresh or frozen mango, chopped and drained

½ c green bell pepper, chopped fine

⅓ c chopped cilantro

Juice of one lime

Mix all ingredients in a large bowl, including the lime juice. Season with sea salt and ground chili pepper to your liking. Allow to marinate in fridge for 30 minutes to an hour. Serve with favorite chips or in romaine lettuce wraps.

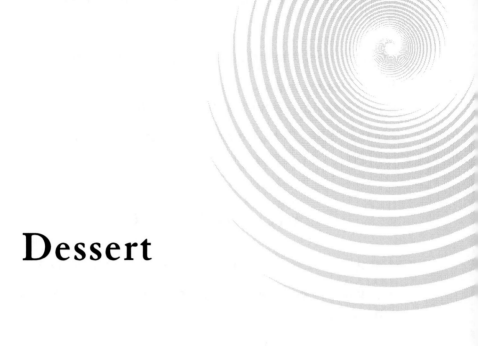

Dessert

APPLESAUCE

8-10 large McIntosh apples*

1 tbsp. cinnamon

1 tsp. cloves

Peel and cut apples into chunks. Try to be mindful while doing this. Seriously, peeling apples can be a total meditation.

Place apple chunks into large pot over medium-low heat. I usually pour about a half cup of water into the pot, so the apples don't burn before they start to break down. Cover pot and allow to sit for 20-30 minutes. Some apples are faster to break down than others. Check in periodically to stir. When the apples are soft and you're able to easily break up the chunks, remove from heat and stir in cinnamon and cloves.

Eat warm or chill in fridge before serving. Great both ways.

*Other apples that work well in applesauce include Brae-burn ,Cortland, Crispin, Fuji, Rome, Ida Red.

Granny Smith do NOT make good applesauce…as I have learned.

APPLE CRISP IN THE RAW

4 large apples, washed well and chopped fine with peels

(Cortland are best because they don't brown as quickly as other apples)

2 tbsp. pure maple syrup

2 tsp. cinnamon

½ tsp nutmeg

juice from half a lemon

¾ c almonds, chopped fine (in processor or by hand)

¾ c pecans

2 tbsp. chia seeds

local honey to drizzle

In a large bowl, mix the chopped apples with the maple syrup, cinnamon, and nutmeg until apples are covered. Add lemon juice and mix again. Pour into serving dish and top with nut mixture. Drizzle honey. Refrigerate for an hour to soften.

Blue Banana Ice Creamy

1 heaping c fresh blueberries

2 frozen bananas

1 tbsp. pure maple syrup or local honey

½ tsp. arrowroot powder

add 2 tbsp non-dairy milk (optional)

Note: You can substitute xantham gum or agar agar flakes for the arrowroot. This ingredient helps to thicken the treat and keeps the ice cream from looking and tasting freezer-burned. Not necessary if you'll be eating right away.

Add the frozen bananas to the high-powered blender or food processor in pieces, then top with blueberries. Blend on high speed until smooth. Add maple syrup and arrowroot and blend again. The mixture will be soft and perfectly fine to eat at this stage, or store in the fridge up to three days. Add milk if necessary to help with blending.

Choco Nut Butter Crunchies

¾ c natural peanut (or other nut) butter (no added sugars)

1 tbsp. local honey

1 c gluten-free (non-GMO) corn flakes, crushed

1½ c dark chocolate chips

Mix nut butter and honey until well combined. Stir in crushed corn flakes. Roll into small balls and place onto wax paper.

Makes 2-4 servings.

1½ c coconut milk (the kind from the can very creamy)

⅓ c chia seeds

½ heaping c of frozen raspberries

1/2 heaping c of frozen blueberries

1 ripe banana, sliced and then quartered pieces

1 heaping tsp. cinnamon

Pour coconut milk into large bowl. Add chia seeds and stir to mix completely. Add frozen fruit and stir again, breaking up any parts frozen together. Allow to sit for ten minutes, then stir again, and break up and parts sticking together. Allow to sit 15 minutes and then add chopped banana and cinnamon. Mix well.

Makes 2-4 servings.

NUT BUTTER CHOCOLATE CHIP TRUFFLES

½ c almond butter (or peanut butter)

½ c sun butter

½ c honey

1 c crushed organic corn flakes or crispy rice cereal

¼ c ground nuts

½ c unsweetened coconut

Mix all ingredients in a medium bowl. Roll into balls. Refrigerate for 30 minutes. Remove from fridge and roll in dark chocolate chips OR shredded coconut, cinnamon, or cacao powder. You decide.

Mom's Peanut Butter Fudge Squares...Redone

Base

½ c rolled oats, ground

1 c peanut butter (no added sugars or hfcs)

1 tbsp. local honey

2 tsp. coconut oil

1 tsp. vanilla extract (pref alcohol-free)

Chocolate Topping

heaping ½ c dark chocolate chips

1 tbsp. coconut oil

Warm honey, vanilla, and coconut oil on top of stove set at medium-low heat. Mix peanut butter with ground oats and add to pot. Mix together with honey/oil blend. Will be somewhat sticky. Spread and flatten with spatula. (I used a loaf pan.) Place in freezer to harden while you prepare topping.

Place coconut oil into pot on low heat. When melted, add dark chocolate chips. Stir and watch carefully so chocolate doesn't burn. When completely melted, remove from eat. Pull peanut butter base from freezer and pour chocolate over base, using spatula to scrape all chocolate from pot. Spread and place back into freezer for an hour.

GOOEY PEANUT BUTTER SQUARES

1 c thick peanut butter

½ c local honey

1¼ c organic non-GMO corn flakes or crispy rice cereal

¼ c ground almonds

Warm peanut butter and honey in pot over stove to low boil. Boil for a few minutes to allow honey to caramelize a bit. Remove from heat. Stir in cereal and nuts. Transfer to an 8×8 baking pan lined with parchment paper. Set in freezer for about 30 minutes. Cut into small squares and serve.

DARK CHOCOLATE ORANGE WAFFLES

Makes 5-6 waffles

1 c full fat coconut milk

1 tsp apple cider vinegar

1 cup brown rice flour

1 cup gluten-free all-purpose flour

½ cup almond or hazelnut flour

2 tsp baking powder

2 cup coconut milk

Grated rind of one large orange (about 2 tbsp)

Juice from one large orange

1 tsp vanilla

1 tsp cardamom

1 tsp salt

¾ cup dark chocolate chips

Start heating waffle iron. Whisk apple cider vinegar into coconut milk. Set aside. Allow to sit as the milk slightly curdles. Combine the dry ingredients and whisk. Add the wet ingredients, including the curdled cup of milk, and stir. Mix in chocolate chips, being careful not to overmix.

Use your waffle iron according to directions.

MOLASSES GINGER COOKIES

Makes 10-12 cookies.

2½ c gluten-free flour*

1 tsp baking powder

1 tsp baking soda

½ tsp salt

1 tbsp powdered ginger

½ c real maple syrup

½ c molasses

½ c organic canola oil

2 tbsp finely grated fresh ginger

If clumpy, sift flour into large bowl and add baking powder, baking soda, salt, and powdered ginger. In a separate bowl, mix maple syrup, molasses, canola oil, and grated ginger. Add the wet ingredients to the dry and stir until just mixed.

Drop by the tablespoon onto a cookie sheet, leaving space between as the cookies will spread. Bake at 350 degrees for about 12 minutes.

*My favorite brand is Cup4Cup

Appendix 1

Herbs for Your Pantry

If you are nursing, pregnant, or on medication, it's a good idea to check with your doctor to see if these herbs are safe for you.

Aloe: used for centuries to treat burns and heal wounds, aloe vera is also full of antioxidants, vitamins, minerals, and compounds with a laxative effect. Add a small piece of the plant leaf to your smoothie.

Anise: reminiscent of black licorice, this herb is known for its benefit for prevention and treatment of flu, cough, and colds. Also helps with digestion and can be used to treat flatulence. Drop an anise star into water and bring to a low boil. Allow to simmer for a few minutes and drink as tea.

Cinnamon: known for its ability to reduce blood pressure and the risk for heart disease, cinnamon makes a great daily addition to your breakfast or dessert in small doses. If using more than once daily or in large amounts, it's best to use Ceylon cinnamon as the standard cassia versions can be toxic to the liver in large amounts.

Lavender: known for its calming properties, sprinkle fresh lavender in the bath or infuse in water and use as a face wash or to cleanse a wound.

Rosemary: carnosol, a compound in rosemary, has cancer-fighting benefits, particularly when it comes to preventing potential harm from carcinogens that form when we grill meat. Use as a marinate or in soups.

Appendix 2

Be an Ingredient Detective

Sadly, food has become political in this country and the bottom line for the food industry often trumps public safety. Being vigilant about the foods we consume is a way to take our power back. Know what you are eating.

Aspartame: Multiple independent studies have found that formaldehyde is formed within cells as the result of aspartame consumption, but more importantly, that this effect is bio-accumulative, meaning more exposure to aspartame increases our risk for cancer. Early studies also find that artificial sweeteners appear to alter the microbiome, potentially leading to weight gain.

149

Food Colors: Some studies have linked certain dye colors-particularly Red 40, Yellow 5 and Yellow 6- to cancer and hyperactivity in children. At the very least, your body doesn't recognize these chemicals as something found in nature so the immune system goes on high alert. If the immune system is constantly activated, our bodies begin to break down.

Monosodium Glutamate: Glutamate is an excitatory transmitter in the brain, and is toxic when present in large amounts. If the blood-brain barrier is in tact in our bodies, then MSG in our foods may not be a concern. Research now indicates that for some people, that barrier is compromised, particularly if the gut microbiome is out of balance. Consuming foods high in MSG, therefore could be a danger and potentially linked to neurological disorders like Parkinson's Disease.

Preservatives: TBHQ, BHA, BHT have all been brought into question as potential carcinogens or as being linked to "abnormal cellular behavior." I do my best to stay away from these. The fewer toxins I put into my body, the better my body can handle the ones I can't avoid.

Appendix 3

Favorite Podcasts

What's a podcast? It's another opportunity to build your tribe, learn something new, and be reinspired to get the most out of your life. I tend to prefer the ones that are less casual conversation and more get-to-the-point kind of format, but search around until you find the ones that resonate most with you. Podcasts are perfect when you're cleaning up the kitchen dishes, stuck in traffic, or folding laundry. There are so many to choose from these days, so ask your friends what they like to listen to, or check out this list below for a starting point.

Happier, with Gretchen Rubin

Hidden Brain

Innovation Hub

Invisibilia

It's Your Health, with Lisa Davis

Jillian Michaels Show

Katy Says

Mindful Spiritual Awakening

Moth Radio Hour

Nutrition Diva

On Being, with Krista Tippett

Radio Lab

Ram Dass Here and Now

Rich Roll

Sessions, with Sean Croxton

TED Radio Hour

Appendix 4

Documentaries To Watch

Documentaries are another great way to empower yourself with knowledge, and I also recommend if you're hoping to get the family on board with new lifestyle choices.

For Nutrition

Fat, Sick & Nearly Dead

Fed Up

Food Matters

Forks Over Knives

Super Size Me

The Future of Food

For General Wellness

Stink!

Unacceptable Levels

For Deeper, Meaningful Inspiration

Awake in the Dream

E-Motion

Finding Joe

Happy

I Am

Kumare

Man on Wire

Searching for Sugar Man

Take it with you